Martin B. Niederle

Neuroendocrine tumours of the digestive tract in Austria

Martin B. Niederle

Neuroendocrine tumours of the digestive tract in Austria

Incidence, diagnosis and treatment

Südwestdeutscher Verlag für Hochschulschriften

Impressum/Imprint (nur für Deutschland/only for Germany)
Bibliografische Information der Deutschen Nationalbibliothek: Die Deutsche Nationalbibliothek verzeichnet diese Publikation in der Deutschen Nationalbibliografie; detaillierte bibliografische Daten sind im Internet über http://dnb.d-nb.de abrufbar.
Alle in diesem Buch genannten Marken und Produktnamen unterliegen warenzeichen-, marken- oder patentrechtlichem Schutz bzw. sind Warenzeichen oder eingetragene Warenzeichen der jeweiligen Inhaber. Die Wiedergabe von Marken, Produktnamen, Gebrauchsnamen, Handelsnamen, Warenbezeichnungen u.s.w. in diesem Werk berechtigt auch ohne besondere Kennzeichnung nicht zu der Annahme, dass solche Namen im Sinne der Warenzeichen- und Markenschutzgesetzgebung als frei zu betrachten wären und daher von jedermann benutzt werden dürften.

Verlag: Südwestdeutscher Verlag für Hochschulschriften GmbH & Co. KG
Dudweiler Landstr. 99, 66123 Saarbrücken, Deutschland
Telefon +49 681 37 20 271-1, Telefax +49 681 37 20 271-0
Email: info@svh-verlag.de

Approved by: Wien, Medizinische Universität, Diss., 2011

Herstellung in Deutschland:
Schaltungsdienst Lange o.H.G., Berlin
Books on Demand GmbH, Norderstedt
Reha GmbH, Saarbrücken
Amazon Distribution GmbH, Leipzig
ISBN: 978-3-8381-2854-2

Imprint (only for USA, GB)
Bibliographic information published by the Deutsche Nationalbibliothek: The Deutsche Nationalbibliothek lists this publication in the Deutsche Nationalbibliografie; detailed bibliographic data are available in the Internet at http://dnb.d-nb.de.
Any brand names and product names mentioned in this book are subject to trademark, brand or patent protection and are trademarks or registered trademarks of their respective holders. The use of brand names, product names, common names, trade names, product descriptions etc. even without a particular marking in this works is in no way to be construed to mean that such names may be regarded as unrestricted in respect of trademark and brand protection legislation and could thus be used by anyone.

Publisher: Südwestdeutscher Verlag für Hochschulschriften GmbH & Co. KG
Dudweiler Landstr. 99, 66123 Saarbrücken, Germany
Phone +49 681 37 20 271-1, Fax +49 681 37 20 271-0
Email: info@svh-verlag.de

Printed in the U.S.A.
Printed in the U.K. by (see last page)
ISBN: 978-3-8381-2854-2

Copyright © 2011 by the author and Südwestdeutscher Verlag für Hochschulschriften GmbH & Co. KG and licensors
All rights reserved. Saarbrücken 2011

Fame or self: Which matters more?
Self or wealth: Which is more precious?
Gain or loss: Which is more painful?
He who is attached to things will suffer much.
He who saves will suffer heavy loss.
A contented man is never disappointed.
He who knows when to stop does not find himself in trouble.
He will stay forever safe.

Tao Te King, XLIV (Translation Chinese - English by Gia-Fu Feng & Jane English, 1972)

Dedicated to my grandparents

Table of Contents

0. Abstracts 11
   0.1 Abstract - English 11
   0.2 Abstract - Deutsch 12

1. Introduction 14

2. Milestones in the elucidation of the gastroentero-pancreatic neuroendocrine system – Historical background 15
   2.1 Pancreas 15
   2.2 Gut 16
   2.3 Inherited tumour syndromes 17

3. The neuroendocrine cell 19
   3.1 Origin and Differentiation 19
      3.1.1 Phylogenetics 20
      3.1.2 Differentiation 21
   3.2 Cell physiology 23
      3.2.1 Identification of neuroendocrine cells 24
      3.2.2 Mechanisms of secretion 26
      3.2.3 The enterochromaffin cell (EC cell) 28
   3.3 Cell types and hormones 30
      3.3.1 Cell types 30
      3.3.2 Enteroendocrine hormones 31
   3.4 Molecular basics of neuroendocrine tumorigenesis 42

4. Neuroendocrine tumours of the gastrointestinal tract 45
   4.1 Histopathological findings 45
      4.1.1 Morphology and microscopy 45
      4.1.2 Immunohistochemistry 46
   4.2 Classification 47
      4.2.1 Former nomenclature and classifications 47
      4.2.2 WHO Classification 2000 47
      4.2.3 WHO Classification 2010 50
      4.2.4 European Neuroendocrine Tumor Society (ENETS) Grading and TNM Classification... 51
      4.2.5 AJCC/UICC TNM-classificiation 51
      4.2.6 Mixed neuroendocrine/non-neuroendocrine tumours ... 52
   4.3 Specific findings at each localisation 52
      4.3.1 Neuroendocrine tumours of the oesophagus 52

4.3.2	Neuroendocrine tumours of the stomach	53
4.3.3	Neuroendocrine tumours of the duodenum	57
4.3.4	Neuroendocrine tumours of the pancreas (PNETs)	61
4.3.5	Neuroendocrine tumours of the jejunum, ileum and Meckel's diverticulum	68
4.3.6	Neuroendocrine tumours of the appendix	72
4.3.7	Neuroendocrine tumours of the colon and rectum	76

4.4 Hereditary tumour syndromes associated with neuroendocrine tumours of the gastrointestinal tract 79

4.4.1	Multiple endocrine neoplasia type 1 (MEN1)	79
4.4.2	Neurofibromatosis type 1 (NF1)	80
4.4.3	Von Hippel-Lindau disease (VHL)	80
4.4.4	Tuberous sclerosis complex	81

4.5 Diagnostic tools 81

| 4.5.1 | Imaging techniques | 81 |
| 4.5.2 | Laboratory tests | 83 |

4.6 Therapeutic options 84

| 4.6.1 | Interventional techniques | 84 |
| 4.6.2 | Medical therapies | 87 |

4.7 Incidence in other countries 89

4.7.1	Godwin II JD - Carcinoid Tumours – An Analysis of 2837 Cases	90
4.7.2	Modlin IM - A 5-Decade Analysis of 13715 Carcinoid Tumors	91
4.7.3	Hemminiki K - Incidence Trends and Risk Factors of Carcinoid Tumors	92
4.7.4	Levi F - Epidemiology of carcinoid neoplasms in Vaud, Switzerland, 1974-97	93

5. Original Research 95

5.1 Aims of the study 95

5.2 Materials and Methods 95

5.2.1	Phase 1: Incidence	96
5.2.2	Phase 2: Clinical evaluation	97
5.2.3	TNM staging and grading based on ENETS definitions	98
5.2.4	Statistical analysis	98
5.2.5	Informed consent	99

5.3 Gastro-entero-pancreatic neuroendocrine tumours - the current incidence and staging based on the WHO and ENETS classification 100

5.3.1	Abstract	100
5.3.2	Introduction	101
5.3.3	Methods	102
5.3.4	Results	105
5.3.5	Discussion	108

  5.3.6 Tables and Figures 115

 5.4 Diagnosis and treatment of gastroenteropancreatic neuroendocrine tumours - Current data on a prospectively collected, retrospectively analyzed clinical multicenter investigation 121

  5.4.1 Abstract 121
  5.4.2 Introduction 122
  5.4.3 Methods 123
  5.4.4 Results 124
  5.4.5 Discussion 128
  5.4.6 Tables 135

6. Conclusions 142
7. References 144
8. Appendices 151

 8.1 Appendix A: List of Austrian institutes of pathology and supporting pathologists 151

 8.2 Appendix B: List of participating clinical institutes and supporting physicians 153

 8.3 Appendix C: Pathological Report Form 156
 8.4 Appendix D: Clinical questionnaire 157
 8.5 Appendix E: Approval 164

9. Lists 166

 9.1 List of abbreviations 166
 9.2 List of tables 169
 9.3 List of figures 171

0. Abstracts

0.1 Abstract - English

Data on the incidence of gastroenteropancreatic neuroendocrine tumors (GEP-NETs) have so far only been obtained retrospectively and are based on inhomogeneous material. In the first part of this analysis a prospective study collecting all newly diagnosed GEP-NETs in Austria during one year was performed. Using the current WHO classification, the TNM staging and Ki67-grading, and the standard diagnostic procedure proposed by the European Neuroendocrine Tumor Society, GEP-NETs from 285 patients (male: 148; female: 137) were recorded. The aim of the second phase of this analysis was to describe "unmasked" clinical symptoms, methods of diagnosis, treatment, and short-term follow-up of gastroenteropancreatic neuroendocrine tumors (GEP-NETs) diagnosed during one year in Austria. 277 patients (excluding those with tumours in the esophagus, gallbladder, a Meckel diverticulum and liver metastasis) were included in the second phase. A standardized questionnaire comprising 50 clinical and biochemical parameters (clinical symptoms, mode of diagnosis, treatment, follow-up) was completed by attending physicians.

The annual incidence rates were 2.51 per 100,000 inhabitants for men, 2.36 for women. The stomach (23%) was the main site, followed by appendix (21%), small intestine (15%) and rectum (14%). Patients with appendiceal tumours were significantly younger than patients with tumours at any other site. 46.0% were classified as benign, 15.4% as uncertain, 31.9% as well-differentiated malignant and 6.7% as poorly differentiated malignant. Patients with benign or uncertain tumours were significantly younger than patients with malignant tumours. Among the malignant tumours of the digestive tract, 1.49% arose from neuroendocrine cells. For malignant gastrointestinal neuroendocrine tumours the incidence was 0.80 per 100,000: 40.9% were ENETS stage I, 23.8% stage II, 11.6% stage III and 23.8% stage IV. The majority (59.7%) were grade 1, 31.2% grade 2 and 9.1% grade 3.

The most common initial symptoms were episodes of abdominal-pain (29.5%), diarrhea (8.7%), weight-loss (7.5%), gastrointestinal-bleeding (5.4%), flushing (3.7%), and bowel-obstruction (3.3%). Overall 48.1% of tumors were diagnosed by endoscopy, 43.7% during surgery, 5% by fine-needle aspiration of the primary or metastases, and 2.5% during autopsy; 44.5% of tumors were not suspected clinically and were diagnosed incidentally during various surgical procedures. Overall 18.7% were removed endoscopically and 67.6% surgically; 13.7% were followed without interventional treatment. Endoscopic/surgical intervention was curative in 81.4% of patients, palliative in 18.6%. At the time of diagnosis, information on metastasis was available in 83.7% with malignant NETs. Lymph node or distant metastases were documented in 74.7%. In 34/176 (19.3%) patients 41 secondary tumors were documented, 78.0% being classified histologically as adenocarcinomas. During a 1-year follow-up 61.5% showed no evidence of disease, 13.5% had stable disease, 16.7% showed progression of disease, and in 8.3% the NET was the cause of death.

0.2 Abstract - Deutsch

Alle bisher gesammelten Daten und Studien über die Inzidenz gastroentero-pankreatischer neuroendokriner Tumoren (GEP-NETs) basieren auf retrospektiv gesammelten Analysen, die auf keiner einheitliche Einteilung der Tumoren beruhen. Aus diesem Grund war es das Ziel dieser Studie, die Inzidenz der GEP-NETs in Österreich basierend auf einem prospektiven Studienprotokoll zu ermitteln. Als Grundlage der Diagnosesicherung und Einteilung dienten die akutelle WHO-Klassifikation sowie das von der European Neudoendocrine Tumour Society (ENETS) erstellte TNM-Staging und Ki67-Grading System. Das Ziel der zweiten Phase der Studie war die Beschreibung der klinischen Symptomatik, der Art der Diagnosestellung, der Behandlung und des kurzfristigen Follow-ups von GEP-NETs im klinischen Alltag in Österreich. 277 Patienten (exkludiert wurden die Tumoren in der Speiseröhre, der Gallenblase, in einem Meckelschen Divertikel sowie die Lebermetastasen) wurden in die zweite Phase eingeschlossen. Ein standardisierter Fragebogen, der ca. 50 Parameter zur Symptomatik, Diagnosemodus, Behandlung, und Follow-up beinhaltete, wurde versandt und von den Behandlern ausgefüllt.

285 Patienten (Männer: 148, Frauen: 137) mit GEP-NETs wurden gesammelt. Die jährliche Inzidenz betrug 2.51 auf 100,000 Einwohner für Männer, und 2.36 für Frauen. Der Magen war die häufigste Lokalisation (23%) gefolgt von Appendix (21%), Dünndarm (15%) und Rektum (14%). Patienten mit Tumoren im Appendix

waren signifikant jünger als Patienten mit Tumoren an anderen Lokalisationen. Die Dignität war bei 46.0% gutartig, 15.4% unklar, 31.9% hoch-differenziert maligne und 6.7% niedrig-differenziert maligne. Unter allen malignen Tumoren im Gastrointestinaltrakt während des Studienzeitraums, entstammten 1.49% von neuroendokrinen Zellen. Die Inzidenz maligner GEP-NETs war 0.80/100,000. Die Einteilung gemäß ENETs Stadien ergab bei 40.9% ENETS Stadium I, 23.8% Stadium II, 11.6% Stadium III und 23.8% Stadium IV. Die Differenzierung der Mehrzahl der Tumoren war Grad 1 (59.7%) gefolgt von 31.2% Grad 2 sowie 9.1% Grad 3.

Die häufigsten Initialsymptome waren unspezifische Bauchschmerzen (29.5%), Durchfall (8.7%), Gewichtsverlust (7.5%), gastrointestinale Blutung (5.4%), Flush (3.7%) und Ileus-Symptomatik (3.3%). Gesamt wurden 48.1% der Tumoren endoskopisch diagnostiziert. Die Diagnose der restlichen erfolgte während Operationen (43.7%), durch Feinnadelpunktion des Tumors oder einer Metastase (5%) oder während der Obduktion (2.5%). 44.5% der Tumoren wurden zufällig entdeckt und wurden während verschiedener Operationen entdeckt. Insgesamt wurden 18.7% endoskopisch und 67.6% operativ entfernt. Follow-up ohne interventionelle Therapie erfolgte in 13.7%. Bei 81.4% der Patienten konnte der Tumor endoskopisch/operativ kurativ entfernt werden, bei 18.6% nur palliativ. Bei 83.7% der malignen Tumore lagen Daten über eine Metastasierung zum Zeitpunkt der Diagnosestellung vor. Davon wurde bei 74.7% Lymphknoten- oder Fernmetastasen diagnostiziert. Bei 34 von 176 (19.3%) der Patienten wurden 41 Begleitkarzinome gezählt, wovon 78.0% histologisch Adenokarzinome waren. Während der 1-jährigen Beobachtungsphase zeigten sich 61.5% der Patienten ohne Hinweis auf einen Tumor, bei 13.5% stabiles Verhalten des Tumors und bei 16.7% eine Tumorprogression. 8.3% verstarben am GEP-NET.

1. Introduction

Neuroendocrine tumours of the gastrointestinal tract are rare neoplasms deriving from the neuroendocrine cells spread along the digestive tract from the oesophagus to the rectum.

These hormone-producing cells were detected about 140 years ago, and about 40 years later it was recognized that tumourous lesions originate from these.

Within the last 100 year a huge number of enteroendocrine hormones and their therapeutic use were detected and tumour associated syndromes caused by the over-production of these hormones were understood. New biochemical tools showed that the origin of neuroendocrine cells is different than thus far predicted and also helped to make the diagnosis of the tumours more accurate. Classification-, staging- and grading systems have been recently developed to optimise the therapeutic management consisting of surgical and medical treatment.

Up to now the incidence of GEP-NETs in Austria has not been assessed because a database addressing neuroendocrine neoplasms was lacking. This special tumour entity is furthermore not recorded adequately in the regular Austrian Cancer database ("Österreichisches Krebsregister"), having no assigned code which differentiates it between the diagnosis of NETs and of other intestinal neoplasms such as adenocarcinomas or lymphomas.

In addition, all other previous international approaches to measure the incidence did not apply the recent classification-systems and little is known about the symptoms and diagnosis in everyday routine.

This book aims to summarize the current knowledge about the origin and hormones of neuroendocrine cells, the current staging- and grading systems and incidence data. The incidence of neuroendocrine tumours of the gastrointestinal tract in Austria is assessed using the recent immunohistochemical tools and applying the current systems for classification, staging and grading. Additionally the practice of diagnosis and treatment in Austria is addressed.

2. Milestones in the elucidation of the gastroenteropancreatic neuroendocrine system – Historical background

In comparison to other endocrine organs, the history of the endocrine system of the digestive tract is rather short. This is, of course, due to the fact that this unique and complex system cannot be investigated or even detected without the help of microscopes. Other endocrine organs were a topic of scientific questioning far earlier. For example, the results of castration were already being described in ancient Egypt and the Bible and in 1841 A.A. Berthold could show that transplantation of the cock's testis can prevent effects of castration. Galen in the 2nd century AD knew about the existence of the pituitary gland and in 1681, J.J. Wepfer suggested that the enlargement of the pituitary gland could be the reason for acromegalic habitus. In 1600 B.C., the Chinese tried to treat goiter with burnt sponge and seaweed and Graves and Basedow described the symptoms of hyperthyroidism around 1800 B.C..[1, 2]

2.1 Pancreas

The history of the neuroendocrine cells of the gastro-enteropancreatic system did not begin until the second half of the 19th century. While the Egyptians were aware of diabetes symptoms, the disease could not be related to an organ until Paul Langerhans from Berlin discovered the islet cells of the pancreas in 1893. Langerhans himself died without understanding the function of these special cells and it was in 1893 when Laguesse proposed that pancreas islet cells produce hormones. The term "hormone" itself was first used by Bayliss and Starling in 1905 after they had detected in 1902 that injection of duodenal mucosa influences the production of pancreatic juice (they detected secretin). After M.A. Lane from Chicago had shown that pancreas islets consisted of different kinds of cells it was J. Homans who concluded that insulin is produced by the ß-cells of the pancreas [1, 2]. The detection of insulin is a fascinating story itself: Despite the fact that it were F.G. Banting (a surgeon!) and J.J.R. MacLeod who received the Noble Prize in Physiology and Medicine in 1923 for the detection of insulin (both of them shared half of the prize with their co-workers C. Best and J. Collip)[3], their work was only further proof of N.C. Paulesco's 1916 experiments which lead to the actual first discovery of insulin. A few years later in 1923, J.R. Murlin and his colleagues detected another hormone which regulates blood glucose levels. They named it glucagon (which was isolated by Staub in 1953). [1, 2]

New diseases could be defined now that the hormone and its producing cells were known. R.M. Wilde and colleagues could show that the symptoms of hyperinsulinism were related to cancer of the islet cells – the insulinoma. Two years later the group of Howland first cured this disease by removing a tumour of the islet cells. [1, 2]

The concept of hyperglucagonemia was described by M.H. McGavran and R.H. Unger in 1966 (USA). Malignant tumors of the alpha-cells were detected. Petersson and Hellman proved that glucagon was produced by the alpha-cells in 1963. [1, 2]

2.2 Gut

Detecting neuroendocrine gut cells and their tumours took even longer than detecting pancreatic cells. It was R.P. Heidenhain in 1867 who first described enterochromaffin cells in gastric mucosa (small granulated cells on the surface of gastric glands). In 1897, Kultschitzky published his work showing the presence of cells in the crypts of the intestinal mucosa which could be stained with silver or chromium salts. However, both failed to elucidate the physiological meaning of these cells. As already mentioned, Bayliss and Starling detected Secretin in 1902 by injecting duodenal mucosa into the bloodstream. Similarly, J.S. Edkins who discovered gastrin in 1906 did this by injecting pyloric mucosa, which resulted in a rise of gastric juice production (this experiment was confirmed by Meydellin in 1913 and R.W. Keeton and F.C. Koch in 1915). [1, 2, 4-6]

S. Oberndorfer was the first to describe tumours of the neuroendocrine gut cells in 1907 (original work [7]). He observed that these tumours grew rather slowly compared to adenocarcinomas and somehow showed a "less malignant" clinical behaviour. He thus introduced the term "Karzinoid" or carcinoma-like which is being used even today. Oberndorfer first thought that these tumours were benign and could not find the cells of origin. In 1914 P. Masson speculated that carcinoid tumours derived from the enteroendocrine cells (he then referred to the cells described by M.C. Ciàccio, who was the first to use the name "enterochromaffin"; original work [8]). In 1928, he published a work describing the major symptoms of carcinoid syndrome (diarrhoea, flush, wheezing, valvular lesions) (original work [9]). In the same year, Ivy and Oldberg described cholezystokinin to influence the contraction and emptying of the gall-bladder. [1, 2, 4-6]

In 1938 the Viennese F. Feyrter, Professor of Pathology in Danzig, Breslau, Göttingen, Graz (after WWII he was also teaching in Vienna and chief of Pathology at Hanusch hospital, was the first to develop the theory of peripheral endocrine glands and of endocrine cells in the GI tract working together as do cells of an organ (original work [10]). [1, 2, 4-6]

After World War II, the story of the gastro-entero-pancreatic systems accelerated. In 1955, R.M. Zollinger and E.H. Ellison described that an islet-cell-tumour was associated with recurring primary peptic ulceration – gastrinoma. Gastrin was isolated by R. Gregory in 1966 (original work [11]). Unger and colleagues detected Enteroglucagon in 1961 and J.C. Brown discovered Motilin in 1966 [1, 2, 4-6].

A.G.E. Pearse, a histochemist, was another scientist who had great impact on the knowledge of GEP neuroendocrine tumours: In 1969 he published the theory of the APUD system (original work [12]). APUD, or amine content, amine-precursor uptake and amino-acid decarboxylase content, sums up all endocrine cells, both in classic endocrine organs and in isolated sites. Most principles of this theory are still accepted today. [1, 2, 4-6]

2.3 Inherited tumour syndromes

Tumour syndromes involving multiple endocrine organs were reported in the second half of the 20th century. Although in 1903 the Viennese pathologist Jacob Erdheim described a case of an acromegalic patient with a pituitary tumour and three enlarged parathyroid glands (original work [13]), it took exactly 50 years for L.O. Underdahl et al to report of eight patients with the combination of pituitary, parathyroid and pancreatic islet adenomas (original work [14]). In 1954, Paul Wermer found that this syndrome was a hereditary syndrome (MEN 1; original work [15]). MEN 2a was detected in 1961 by J.H. Sipple (original work [16]) and E.D. Williams described MEN 2b in 1966 (original work [17]). The term "multiple endocrine neoplasia" itself was introduced by A.L. Steiner in 1968 (original work [18]). [19]

3. The neuroendocrine cell

3.1 Origin and Differentiation

The last three decades brought a lot of new insights into the origins and the mechanisms of neuroendocrine differentiation in the gastrointestinal system. Former concepts could be refuted by sophisticated experiments that were made possible by new scientific technologies, especially in genetics. [20, 21]

In 1928, P. Masson was the first to propose that gastroentero-pancreatic neuroendocrine cells were of neural origin and thus deriving from ectoderm (original work [9]) as did Sunder-Plassmann in 1939. And one year later, Altmann proposed that these cells might be chemosensors derived from ectoderm (original work [22]). Together with the APUD-theory, Pearse stated in 1969, that neuroendocrine cells were both derived from neural crest and connected to the nervous system and thus acted as the endocrine division of the neuronal network, modulating faster signals (original work [12]). His chicken embryo studies apparently supported his theory although he was never able to prove it absolutely.[20, 21]

Pearse's theory still holds true for some cells of the APUD-systems, e.g. the thyroidal C-cell, but in 1963, A. Andrew and colleagues could show for the first time, that the enterochromaffin cells' stem cells are NOT neuronal. She eliminated or marked the neuroectodermal cells that were thought to be the source and could show that they could not be the origin of both pancreatic and intestinal neuroendocrine cells. As a consequence, Pearse adapted his theory and then proposed that neuroendocrine-programmed ectoblast cells are the origin. This new theory could not be refuted at first, but lineage-tracing experiments helped to find the true source cells of the gastrointestinal neuroendocrine cells (cf. [20, 21]):

All epithelial cell lineages in the gastrointestinal tract derive from a single stem cell and are clonal populations [23]. Even after destruction of intestinal crypts by radiation, for example, a single stem cell can regenerate crypts which include all epithelial cells (enterocytes, goblet-cells, Paneth cells, enteroendocrine cells). Thus, it was proposed that these stem cells (clearly of endodermal origin) are the source cells for neuroendocrine cells in the gut and this theory was proved by Ponder et colleagues showing that all cell lineages in a crypt definitely derive from the same stem cells [24].

Further experiments by Thompson (using XX/XY chimeric mice [25]) and Novelli (using cells of a patient suffering from familial adenomatous polyposis with chimeric X0/XY genotype [26] and cells of G6PD defective heterozygous Sardinan females [27]) showed that all cells in a Lieberkühn crypt are monoclonal and that there are no mixed crypts. Most recently, McDonald and colleagues used cells with mitochondrial mutations (cytochrom c oxidase deficiency = cox). Cox-deficient cells destroy other cells in a crypt totally occupying the crypt. As a consequence the crypt then contains all cell lineages and all of them (including neuroendocrine cells) are cox-deficient [28].

These experiments clearly show that neuroendocrine cells of the gastrointestinal tract do not derive from the neural crest and thus are not ectodermal of origin but endodermal. [20, 21]

3.1.1 Phylogenetics

Traces of endocrine cells (see **Figure 1**) in the intestinal tract affiliated with neurons can be traced back to cnidarian species (simple animals; e.g. jellyfish, corals, anemones, hydras). In the Hydra's (dipoblastic animals = having two germ layers, endoderm and ectoderm) digestive tract, neurosecretory cells can be found. These produce peptides such as cholezystokinin, bombesin, and calcitonin etc. These cells are not the evolutionary predecessors of mammalian enteroendocrine cells because they are bipolar sensory neurons but they can be considered functional precursors. [29]

Endoderm derived cells expressing peptides can be found in all bilaterian organisms exhibited thus far. These cells do not derive from neuronals cells, although in Platyhelminthes (flatworms) both types of cells (neurosecretory and "endocrine") can be found. [29]

In phylum Protostomes, the gut begins to specialise along its course as do enteroendocrine cells. The cells begin to accumulate and sometimes form groups in the submucosal tissue. In snails and bivalve species, dispersed cells with immunoreactivity for insulin-like peptides are detected for the first time.

In Deuterostomes, the development of regional specification and formation proceeds and in jawless fish, not only the pituitary and the thyroid can be found but also an endocrine pancreas. In embryogenesis of jawless fish, it is observed for the first time that enteroendocrine cells migrate out of the gut to form an organ. [29]

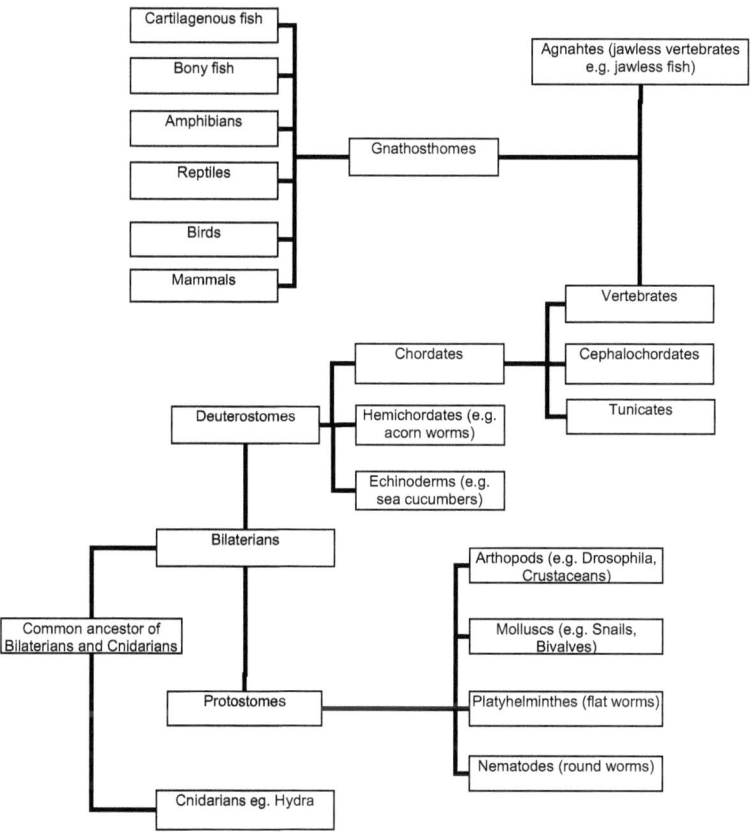

Figure 1 - Schematic and simplified phylogenetic tree adapted from S. Leach [29]

3.1.2 Differentiation

Some important mechanisms of differentiation in gastrointestinal neuroendocrine cells are known but this topic has only been elucidated rudimentarily. As mentioned above, intestinal NE-cells derive from a multi-potent stem cell, which is the source for all 4 epithelial cell types: Enterocytes (for absorption), goblet cells (producing mucous), Paneth cells and enteroendocrine cells. The crypt of Lieberkühn is the functional anatomical unit of the small intestine and every cell of a single crypt is a monoclonal daughter cell of75 a single source-cell at the base of the crypt. Starting there, cells move during multiple amplification cycles to the top of the villus and meanwhile differentiate into one of the four "specialised" cells (except for Paneth cells which do not move upwards to the top but downwards into the submucosal layer). In addition to this process of differentiation, there is another along the intestine from duodenum to colon – multiple factors are involved in the differentiation into the multiple types of neuroendocrine cells (EC cells, G cells, L cells etc.) in the diverse parts of the gut. [30-33]

Some genes and transcription factors are known: the locoregional differentiation is influenced by homeotic genes (hox-genes; e.g. pdx1). These genes originally found in drosophila flies are known to determine the placement and formation of segments of the body. For example, mice lacking the pdx1 gene homozygous do not develop a pancreas at all, whereas isolated pdx1-inactivation in beta-cells leads to insulin deficiency. [30-33]

The other differentiation process from endodermal stem cell to endocrine cell is induced by activation of genes that are also important for the differentiation of neuronal cells and glia cells, e.g. Neurogenins (especially Neurogenin 3, Ngn3), Math1 and Neuro D. These genes are members of the bHLH (basic helix loop helix) transcription factor family that bind to cis-acting regulatory DNA elements, which in turn activate RNA polymerase 2 and thus RNA transcription. Mice experiments have shown that knock-out Ngn3 -/- mice do not develop pancreatic islet cells at the embryonic stage or later. The animals die shortly after birth of severe diabetes. Further studies have shown that Ngn3 is mandatory for most neuroendocrine cells, especially in pancreatic islets but some cells in the stomach (EC cells, ECL cells) develop even in Ngn3 mutant mice. [30-33]

Further genes involved in enteroendocrine differentiation are PAX genes (= paired box genes; family of transcription factors with paired domain and usually a partial or complete homeodomain). Pax mutations (Pax4, Pax6) lead to absent islet alpha and/or beta cells and to reduced number of endocrine cells in stomach and duodenum as well. [30-33]

Another interesting phenomenon in enteroendocrine differentiation is lateral inhibition. Endodermal stem cells express Notch, a transmembran receptor which, via its intracellular component, is able to alter gene expression. If neurogenin or NeuroD is activated in one of these cells, the cell also expresses Delta, a transmembrane ligand. Delta binds to the Notch receptor of the neighbour cells which activates expression of Hes1, also a member of the bHLH-family. Hes1 represses transcriptional processes and thus inhibits expression of neurogenin or NeuroD in a cell with Notch-activation by Delta-ligand. Thus, cells inhibit their neighbours to differentiate in the same way. Hes1-/- knock out mice show an increase in numbers of many enteroendocrine cell lineages, whereas the pancreas itself is hypoplastic. [30-33]

These are together only some details of enteroendocrine differentiation. They show the complexity of these mechanisms but leave us far from a complete understanding.

3.2 Cell physiology

As explained above, neuroendocrine tumours and neuronal cells are of different origin. Nonetheless they share a lot of characteristics and often behave similarly. [34, 35] Neurons and neuroendocrine cells both have a polarised membrane orientation, two separate regulated secretory pathways (and one not-regulated, constitutive way) and share neurotransmitter-synthesizing enzymes and neural cell adhesion molecules (e.g. N-CAM). In addition, both of them produce peptides and amino acid neurotransmitters that are stored in membrane-coated vesicles or granules. These are secreted upon second messenger signals activated by a(n) (external) stimulus. [34, 35]

The products of neuroendocrine cells, hormones and neurotransmitters, act paracrine on neighbouring tissues, endocrine on distant tissues and sometimes autocrine on the secreting cell itself. All different types of these cells form a network which complexly regulates, adapts and tunes mechanisms of secretion, absorption, motility and mucosal cell proliferation in the gastrointestinal tract. Additionally, there is evidence that they may interact with the immune system too, influencing the immune-barrier control in the gut. [34, 35]

3.2.1 Identification of neuroendocrine cells

By microscopy, neuroendocrine cells of the intestinal tract are shown to be clear, small cells in comparison to to enterocytes [34]. They can be found either in the mucosa with contact to the gut lumen (open-type cells) or under a layer of enterocytes without any connection to the lumen (closed-type cells). They sometimes form groups in the intestine whereas in the pancreas these cells can always be found accumulated together in groups, the so-called Langerhans islets [29]. However, in the pancreas, they are also positioned throughout the exocrine ducts. Neuroendocrine cells usually have a clear cytoplasma in in which granules can be found using special staining techniques. Before immunohistochemistry was available, staining methods for detecting neuroendocrine cells had basically been reduced to silver (silver nitrate) and chromium (potassium dichromate) impregnation techniques as neuroendocrine cells are able to take up and reduce silver and chromium ions in the absence or presence of reducing agents (Masson-Fontana stain; Grimelius stain). This is the reason why the cells were called argentaffin or enterochromaffin cells. [34, 35]

Nowadays specific antibodies against target antigens (proteins) can be produced and combined with either enzymes or fluorophores to make them visible (principle of immunohistochemistry). Thus we are able to look for distinct markers in cells to classify them precisely. [34, 35]

In neuroendocrine cells these target proteins are markers of neuronal differentiation. As mentioned above GI-neuroendocrine cells derive from a multipotent endodermal stem cell and differentiate by activation of genes also involved in the differentiation of neurons – actually, neuronal and neuroendocrine cells share a lot of specific proteins. These can either be found in the cell's cytosol or in the secretory granules or are adhesion molecules. [34, 35]

Cytosolic markers

Neuron specific enolase (NSE): NSE is a phosphopyruvate dehydratase, which is involved in glycolysis, and found mainly in neurons and neuroendocrine cells.
Protein gene product 9.5 (PGP 9.5): PGP 9.5 is an ubiquitin-hydrolase and predominantely expressed in neuronal tissues and neuroendocrine cells. [34, 35]

Granular markers

Chromogranin A (CgA): CgA is a member of the granin-family (chromogranin/secretogranin) and found in secretory granules, mainly in large density core vesicles (LDCVs) of neurons and neuroendocrine cells (see further details below)

Synaptophysin (Syn): Syn is a synaptic vesicle protein mainly in small synaptic vesicles, found in many neuroendocrine cells and neurons.

Vesicular monoamine transporter 1 and 2 (VMAT1/2): VMAT is an ATP-dependent transporter protein which "fills" monoamine-peptides into membrane-coated vesicles (secretory vesicles). VMAT1 is found in serotonin-producing EC-cells whereas VMAT2 is present in Histamin-producing ECL-cells and pancreatic islet-cells.

Protein 55: Protein 55 is an acidic protein of the granin family in LDCVs.

Synaptic vesicle protein 2 (SV2): SV2 is a membrane glycoprotein found in secretory vesicles of neurons and neuroendocrine cells. [34, 35]

Cell adhesion molecules

Neuronal cell adhesion molecules (N-CAM): N-CAM are important molecules located on the surface of neurons and neuroendocrine cells. [34, 35]

Specific markers

Approximately 14 different types of neuroendocrine cells in the gastrointestinal tract are known and produce specific peptide hormones and biogenic amines (see 3.3). These cells can be differentiated by detecting specific peptide-products or with the use of electron microscopy as the granules contained in a cell differ by shape, size and electron density. The granules' appearance is often not sufficient to specify cell type : On one hand, there are granules that look the same but may contain multiple hormones (e.g. in EC cells and L cells), on the other, one hormone can have differently shaped granules in the same cell type. Thus, only specific peptide profiles ascertained by staining techniques can differentiate the types of enteroendocrine cells. [34, 35]

3.2.2 Mechanisms of secretion

There are two fundamental mechanisms of secretion: constitutive secretion and regulated secretion

Constitutive secretion can be found in every cell. Vesicles leave the cell continuously without any external stimulus. This mechanism is used both for secretion of proteins such as albumins, immunglobulins or elements of the cell membrane (such as receptors, antigens, etc.) but also for exocytosis of molecules that are not needed anymore in the cell. [34, 35]

Conversely, regulated secretion is a specific feature in secretory cells such as endocrine cells or neurons. It is triggered by an external stimulus which causes an intracellular second messenger signal. This signal leads to exocytosis of stored vesicles. [34, 35]

The first step in protein secretion is always protein synthesis. Specific genes are express depending on the cell's biological program (cell type). After gene transcription to m-RNA and activation of ribosomes, polypeptide chains are synthesized at the rough endoplasmatic reticulum (RER – process of translation). This process depends on sufficient support of molecules needed, such as glucose and amino acids. Therefore, neuroendocrine cells possess various specific transporters in the plasma membrane, vesicles, endosomes and mitochondria which transport specific molecules against concentration gradients into the cell compartment where they are needed (e.g. VMAT). These transporters are important for diagnosis and perhaps treatment of neuroendocrine tumours. The polypeptide-chains produced are transported into the Golgi apparatus, where they are further processed by enzymes (e.g. proprotein-convertase 1, 2 and 3 [PC1, 2 and 3]; carboxpeptidase E) and finished by defined proteolytic steps. They are then packed with other proteins into vesicles and sorted. The chromogranin-secretogranin family plays a very important role in intracellular transport and sorting of proteins. Multiple hormones such as chromogranin A, chromogranin B or secretogranin 2-6 belong to the granin family. They are soluble secretory proteins and consist of 180-700 amino acids. Chromogranins have an affinity to Ca and low pH – both can be found in the Golgi apparatus. They accumulate and bind there to specific proteins (such as serotonin, histamin and others) thereby separating molecules for regulated secretion from others that are secreted continuously. Experiments with antisense RNA against CgA-RNA showed that without CgA, regulated secretion is almost completely inhibited. [34, 35]

Besides, chromogranins themselves have specific binding sites for endopeptidases and are precursors of bioactive peptides [36] (see below).

Vesicles

As mentioned above, some of the vesicles continuously pass and bud from the Golgi apparatus and leave the cell without any control (constitutive pathway). Others are stored in the cytoplasma and are released upon cell stimulation (regulated pathway). Constitutive vesicles and regulated vesicles can only be differentiated with specific staining techniques. Regulated vesicles can be subdivided into two different groups: Large dense core vesicles (LDCV) and small synaptic vesicles (SSV; alternative name: synaptic-like microvesicles [SLMV]). [34, 35]

LDCVs have a diameter of approximately 100-400nm (detectable under electron microscope) and contain mainly polypeptides. Their immunohistochemical marker is chromogranin A. [34, 35]

SSVs are smaller than LDCVs and have a lower molecular weight. They mainly contain neurotransmitters, which often are produced within (via glutamic acid decarboxylase, cholinacetyl transferase, neuronal NO synthetase etc.). Their immunohistochemical marker is synaptophysin. [34, 35]

Exocytosis

Another interesting issue is the docking and fusion of secretory vesicles. These processes have been closely investigated in neuronal cells and there is much evidence that mechanisms are very similar in neuroendocrine cells. Both the vesicle and the membrane contain a SNARE-complex (Soluble NSF-associated attachment receptor). The vesicle-SNARE complex (v-SNARE) consists of the membrane proteins synaptobrevin and synaptotagmin. Synaptotagmin is activated by increasing Ca concentrations in the cell and changes its conformation – this leads to binding of the v-SNARE to the target-SNARE complex (t-SNARE) complex (syntaxin, SNAP25). This process requires the cytosolic factors NSF (N-ethylmaleimide-sensitive factor) and SNAPs (soluble NSF-associated proteins). It is known that tetanus toxin and botulinum inhibit vesicle docking via proteolysis of synaptobrevin, SNAP 25 and syntaxin, which might be of therapeutic interest [37, 38]

Receptors

There are three major types of cell receptors in neuroendocrine cells: G-protein coupled receptors, ligand directed channels (ion-gated receptor) and receptors with tyrosine kinase activity. Secretion is mainly initiated by Ca influx into the cell which activates enzymes (Protein kinases, synthetases), proteins involved in vesicle movement (e.g. actin) and others. There is also evidence that subunits of G proteins play an important roll in intracellular vesicle transport binding directly to SSVs and LDCVs. G protein coupled receptors can also inhibit secretion by lowering the calcium concentration in the cell (e.g. somatostatin receptors via Gi-receptors). [35]

3.2.3 The enterochromaffin cell (EC cell)

The enterochromaffin cell is the most frequently occurring endocrine cell in the gastrointestinal tract. Its function should be summarized briefly:
The cell is localised in the gut mucosa, mainly as an open-type cell, from the stomach to the anus. Although its shape is rather variable, the polarized membrane usually has a microvilli-tuft on one side, which reaches in to the lumen of the gut. The other side reaches the submucosa and has multiple dendritic processes that have cell-to-cell contacts to smooth muscle cells, neurons (enteric neuron system ENS; central nervous system CNS), other neuroendocrine cells, enterocytes, goblet cells and very

likely immunocytes as well. The cell stores secretory vesicles mainly at the base and these are released upon various stimuli. Hormone exocytosis can be initiated by luminal contents such as nutrients (glucose, aromatic amino acids etc.) which pass the cell's microvilli and by bile salt exposition. Recent studies show that not only the EC-cell but most other open-type neuroendocrine cells in the gastrointestinal tract have special receptors on their microvilli reaching the intestinal lumen. These receptors are very similar to the taste receptors on the tongue and belong to the family of T1R and T2R receptor (G-protein coupled receptors) [39]. Thus different tastes (different nutritional components) cause different actions in the gut, which is not only important for digestion but also for defence against toxins and micro-organisms [40]. The cell is furthermore influenced by the central and enteric nervous system via α- and β-adrenergic neurons, receptors for PACAP (pituitary adenylat cyclase activating peptide; found in CNS as neurohormone, neuromodulator, neurotransmitter but also as hormone and immunmodulator), that stimulate exocytosis too. Some other agents inhibit release of vesicles: Acetylcholin (via Muscarin-receptors), GABA (gamma amino butyric acid; $GABA_A$-receptor) and somatostatin. Autocrine effects via 5-HT-receptors (both stimulating and inhibiting) are very likely. Additionally on the cell's surface, receptors for various growth factors (endothelic growth factor EGF, fibroblastic growth factor FGF etc.) can be found that modulate genetic programs (growth, repair, apoptosis). [39]

The EC cell's granules contain the following proteins: Serotonin, melatonin, substance P and guanylin. Serotonin stimulates both bicarbonate secretion in the duodenum and pancreatic secretion. It also stimulates proliferation of endothelial cells and interstitial cell's of Cajal (enteric pacemaker cells). Serotonin is also a neurotransmitter and thereby regulates gastric motility and peristalsis in the whole intestine. Melatonin influences bicarbonate secretion via vagal and sympathetic stimulation. Substance P activates smooth muscle cells and the interstitial cells of Cajal. Guanylin is involved in electrolyte homeostasis in the intestinal epithelium and can also regulate renal tubular function. Additionally, guanylin has a direct stimulating influence on goblet cells. [39]

Together, the EC cell connects and coordinates different cell systems in the intestine. It is a kind of chemosensor, sensing and reacting to luminal contents by stimulation of the enteric and central nervous systems. It thereby coordinates movement of neighbouring sectors in the intestine and furthermore regulates secretion into the gut lumen and perhaps connects the immunsystem to other systems and thus has an impact on the gut's immune barrier. [39]

3.3 Cell types and hormones

3.3.1 Cell types

Approximately 14 different endocrine cell types can be distinguished in the gastrointestinal tract including those in the pancreas. As mentioned above, they can only be typified with immunohistochemical stainings for special peptides. A single cell type can produce multiple biologically active peptides. [33, 34]

Table 1 summarises the most important types and their products.

Cell type	Localisation in gastrointestinal tract	Main product
A cells	Islets of pancreas	Glucagon
B cells	Islets of pancreas	Insulin
D cells	Stomach, duodenum, small intestine, colon	Somatostatin
EC cells (enterochromaffin cells)	Stomach, duodenum, small intestine, colon, rectum	Serotonin
ECL cells	Stomach	Histamin
G cells	Stomach and duodenum	Gastrin
I cells	Duodenum, jejunum	Cholecystokinin
K cells	Duodenum and proximal jejunum	GIP
L cells	Ileum, colon, rectum	GLP-1, GLP-2, PYY
M cells	Duodenum, proximal jejunum	Motilin
N cells	Small intestine (ileum)	Neurotensin
P/D1 cells	Stomach, duodenum, jejunum	Ghrelin
PP cells	Islets of pancreas	Pancratic polypeptide
S cells	Duodenum, proximal jejunum	Secretin

Table 1 - GI neuroendocrine cell types, their localisations and main products (after [33, 34])

3.3.2 Enteroendocrine hormones

Several biologically active proteins are known to be produced in the gastrointestinal tract, not all of them acting as "hormones" in the original sense. They are secreted from closed-type cells into the circulation acting as "classical" hormones (endocrine) or are released in the neighbouring tissue (paracrine). Because these peptides can also stimulate neurons, they can be subdivided into hormones and neurotransmitters – some are hormones in the gastrointestinal-tract but neurotransmitters in the CNS and some function as a hormone and as a neurotransmitter in the gastrointestinal tract (action on non-neuronal cells AND nerves; e.g. cholecystokinin). [33, 41]

Open-type cells secret their products into the gut lumen also, thereby influencing the mucosal cells with contact to the lumen. Most of enteroendocrine peptides are also known to have an autocrine activity, mainly for an auto-feedback mechanism for inhibiting their own release. [33, 41]

The genes encoding for many of these proteins are highly conserved – as mentioned above some of them can already be found in primitive species. Furthermore one gene can be transcribed into many different peptides via different splicing and different enzymatic modification (e.g. calcitonin-gene-related peptide [CRGP] and calcitonin; glucagon and glucagon-like-Protein 1 and 2). Additionally, peptides often have clearly evident similarities in their amino-acid-structure, such as gastrin and cholecystokinin or VIP and secretin despite their different effects. [33, 41]

Together, gastrointestinal hormones are important for digestion, coordinating gastrointestinal movement and secretion. They influence distant tissues (liver, muscles and fat tissue) to react on resorbed nutritional components and also control processes in the central nervous systems, such as hunger and satiety[42]. Additionally gastrointestinal hormones may be influencing inflammation processes in the gut[43]. Some of these peptides also stimulate growth and renewal of all mucosal cell types. [33, 41]

Most neuroendocrine peptides have their own cell-membrane-bound – receptor that can either have stimulating or inhibiting effects. As mentioned above, these receptors are either G-protein coupled receptors, ligand directed channels (ion-gated receptor) or receptors with tyrosine kinase activity. In the future, specific receptors may be important both in diagnostics and therapy. [33, 41]

In the following section, the most important and investigated peptides are presented and subdivided into those mainly with hormonal actions and those predominantly acting as neurotransmitters.

Endocrine-acting peptides

Serotonin (5-HT3)

Localisation and production: Serotonin is produced in the EC cells which can be found throughout the gastrointestinal lumen from stomach to anus.
Structure: It is a biogenous amine produced out of the amino acid tryptophan (taken up directly from the gut lumen) via a hydroxylase- and a decarboxylase-step. It is degraded by a monoamine-oxidase (MAO) and aldehyd-decarboxylase into 5-Hydrox-inodol-acetic-acid. Nearly all body serotonin is produced in the gastrointestinal tract.
Stimulation of secretion: Luminal stimulation: Mechanical, chemical (acidification), nutritional components, neuronal (from CNS via parasympathetic nerves and from enteric nervous system [ENS])
Inhibition of secretion: Somatostatin, beta-adrenergic nerves
Actions: Regulates bicarbonate, chloride and water secretion, mucus production, peristalsis as well as exocrine pancreatic secretion, potential pro-inflammatory effects. [33, 39, 41, 43]

Insulin

Insulin is clearly the most well-known gastrointestinal hormone. Its qualities should therefore be summarized only briefly.
Localisation and production: Insulin is produced out of preproinsulin of pancreatic beta cells (B-cells) which is then further processed by proprotein convertase 1 and 2 to proinsulin.
Structure: Insulin consists of 51 aminoacids after removal of the c-peptide via carboxypeptidase E.

Stimulation of secretion: Glucose is of course the most important stimulating factor for insulin release. Under physiological conditions, a rise in blood glucose concentration results in a dose-dependent rise of insulin secretion. The same amount of intravenous glucose infusion and oral glucose uptake results in a different amount of insulin release. Intravenous glucose stimulates the ß-cells less than oral glucose. This effect is called the "incretin-effect" and is mainly caused by the enteroendocrine hormones GIP and GLP-1 (see below). Amino acids and to less extent fatty acids, also stimulate insulin release. Other stimulatory hormonal factors are Glucagon, but also VIP, GRP and PACAP via parasympathetic stimulation. ß-cells can also be directly stimulated by parasympathetic nerves. There is also a periodic oscillation in the ß-cell insulin release.

Inhibition of secretion: Somatostatin and α-adrenergic receptors

Actions: Regulates glucose homeostasis by lowering blood glucose via stimulation of glucose uptakein muescle and fat cells, and inhibition of gluconeogenesis and glycogenolysis in liver cells, insulin further stimulates glycogen synthesis in muscle and liver and fatty acid uptake and triglyceride synthesis in liver and adipose tissue.
[33, 41, 44]

Gastrin

Localisation and production: Gastrin is produced in the G cells mainly localised in the antrum of the stomach and the upper small intestine, but also in the CNS.

Structure: There are 3 major forms, cleaved from a 101 amino-acid prohormone: G14, G17 and G34 (highest concentration in circulation). The gastrin activity is mediated mainly via cholecystokinin-B/gastrin-receptor (gastrin and cholecystokinin have the same 5 amino acids at their C-terminal end – so there are receptors that are stimulated by both hormones)

Stimulation of secretion: Amino acids and proteins in stomach lumen, distension of stomach. Neuronal: Vagal stimulation (acetylcholine), ß-adrenergic. Hormonal: Gastrin releasing peptide (GRP);

Inhibition of secretion: gastric pH < 3, somatostatin, calcitonin-gene related peptide

Actions: Stimulation of H+-ione release from gastric parietal cells, stimulation of histamin-release from ECL-cells, stimulation of pepsin and intrinsic-factor release from chief cells, trophic effects on gastric mucosa. [33, 41]

Cholecystokinin (CCK)

Localisation and production: Cholecystokinin is produced in the I cells, mainly in the duodenum and upper part of the jejunum. CCK can be found as a neurotransmitter in the nervous system in the CNS in the hypothalamus, cerebral cortex and neurohypophysis and also in the ENS (large intestine).
Structure: There are many forms of CCK including CCK-8 (mainly in CNS), CCK-22, CCK-33 (predominant in circulation), CCK-39 and CCK-58. There are two receptors CCK-A, mainly in the gastrointestinal tract and CCK-B, which is predominant in the CNS but also found in the gastrointestinal tract (Gastrin is a high affinity ligand to CCK-B-receptors).
Stimulation of secretion: Digests nutrients in the upper part of the small intestine (in particular fatty acids, L-amino-acids). Hormonal: Gastrin-releasing peptide.
Inhibition of secretion: Trypsin, bile salts, somatostatin
Actions: Empties the gall bladder. Inhibits gastric emptying (via stimulating effect on gastric D-cells). Stimulates pancreatic endocrine cells. Possibly effects satiety via efferent nerves. Effects growth on both pancreatic acini and islets (in rodents). [33, 41, 45]

Secretin

Localisation and production: It is secreted by S cells localised in the duodenum and proximal jejunum but also found in the CNS and fetal pancreas.
Structure: Secretin is a 27-amino-acid peptide
Stimulation of secretion: pH in duodenum <4.5 (gastric acids), fatty acids and bile salts in duodenum
Inhibition of secretion: Somatostatin

Actions: Rises pH in duodenum by bicarbonate secretion of pancreas, liver and Brunner's duodenal glands. Augments pancreatic enzyme production and secretion. Inhibits gastric movement and acid release, stimulates pepsinogen in stomach. Stimulates gallbladder. [33, 41]

Gastric inhibitory polypeptide = Glucose dependent insulinotropic polypeptide (GIP)

Localisation and production: GIP is produced in the K cells mainly in the duodenum and upper jejunum
Structure: 42-amino acid peptide
Stimulation of secretion: Nutritional components (fatty acids, glucose, amino acids)
Inhibition of secretion: unknown
Actions: Acts as an incretin: stimulates pancreatic B-cells to produce and secrete insulin (only in supra-normal levels). Effect on gastric motility (acceleration of gastric emptying) is possible but under discussion. [33, 41, 46]

Glucagon

Localisation and production: Glucagon is a 29-amino acid peptide produced mainly in the pancreatic A cells. It is also found in the brain, mainly in the brain stem and hypothalamus.
Structure: It consists of 29-amino acid peptide and belongs to the family of proglucagon-derived peptides (PGDPs) that originate from the 180 amino-acid Proglucagon (others: GLP-1, GLP-2, enteroglucagon = glicentin, oxyntomodulin)
Stimulation of secretion: Hypoglycemia, catecholamines, adrenergic stimulation, Cholezystokinin
Inhibition of secretion: Somatostatin, Insulin
Actions: Crucial for glucose homeostasis by increasing glycogenolysis and gluconeogensis. [33, 41]

Glucagon-like Protein 1 and 2 (GLP-1, GLP-2)

Localisation and production: GLP-1 and GLP-2 are other members of the PGDP-family and are produced in intestinal L cells.

Structure: GLP-1 is a 30 amino-acid protein. GLP-2 consists of 33-amino-acids. Their actions are mediated via special GLP-receptors. GLPs are inactivated via dipeptidyl-peptidase 4 (DPP4).

Stimulation of secretion: Ingestion of food, particularly Glucose resorption

Inhibition of secretion: unknown

Actions: GLP-1: Increases insulin release and insulin gene expression. Lowers glucagon secretion. Stimulates pancreatic islet growth; inhibits B-cell apoptosis. Inhibits gastric emptying. Influences hunger (via receptors in the CNS). GLP-2: Trophic factor on crypt cell proliferation. [33, 41, 42, 47]

Enteroglucagon = Glicentin

Localisation and production: Enteroglucagon is also produced in the L cells

Structure: It consists of 69 amino-acids

Stimulation of secretion: Released upon nutritional contents in the gut lumen (fatty acids)

Inhibition of secretion: Somatostatin

Actions: Enteroglucagon is thought to have trophic effects on intestinal cell proliferation [33, 41, 47]

Oxyntomodulin

Localisation and production: Found basically in the small intestine

Structure: Oxyntomodulin shares the amino acid sequence with glucagon and has an additional octapeptid. It is known to be effective via glucagon receptors (with lower affinity).

Stimulation of secretion: unknown

Inhibition of secretion: unknown

Actions: Inhibiting acid secretion in the stomach, Potentially oxyntomodulin administered subcutaneously can reduce body weight. [33, 41, 42, 48]

Motilin

Localisation and production: It is produced in M-cells predominantly in the small intestine and to a lesser degree in the large intestine but also in the gall bladder and biliary tract.
Structure: Motilin is a peptide consisting of 22-amino-acids and belongs to the ghrelin peptide family
Stimulation of secretion: Gastric distension, duodenal acidification, vagal stimulation, periodic release every 90-120 minutes
Inhibition of secretion: Somatostatin, pancreatic polypeptide (PP)
Actions: Initiates phase 3 contractions (= Peristaltic contraction every 90-120 minutes; cleaning gut lumen, avoiding bacterial overgrowth) of the migrating motor complex (MMC). Erythromycin interacts with Motilin-receptors (used for prokinetic effects). Stimulates gastric and pancreatic enzyme release, contraction of gallbladder, sphincter Oddi and oesophageal sphincter. [33, 41, 49]

Somatostatin (SS)

Localisation and production: It is produced in cells distributed all over the gastrointestinal tract, found especially in the D-cells of pancreatic islets. Somatostatin is also a neurostransmitter in the CNS. It has a short have-life. Longer-acting syntetic somatostatin-analogues (octreotide and lanreotide) are important for diagnostic and therapeutic aspects in neuroendocrine tumours. Five somatostatin-receptors are known thus far (SSTR1-5; G-protein-coupled receptors). SSTR2 is expressed most often in gastrointestinal neuroendocrine tumours
Structure: Two different forms of somatostatin are known thus far: SS-14 and SS-28. The active component of somatostatin consists of a beta-turn formed by 4 aminoacids.
Stimulation of secretion: nutritional components (fat, proteins), low-PH, GIP, CCK, secretin, stimulation via CNS

Inhibition of secretion: Opioids

Actions: Inhibition of both endocrine and exocrine secretion in the gastrointestinal tract (reduced calcium influx, inhibition of adenyl-cyclase activity), inhibition of intestinal motilily, inhibition of growth hormone and thyrotropin-release (inhibiting cell growth). [33, 41, 50]

Neurotensin

Localisation and production: Neurotensin is produced in N-cells (ileums, lesser extent jejunum), CNS, heart, adrenal gland, pancreas and respiratory tract.
Structure: It consists of 13 amino-acids and is related to Neuromedin N (same precursor molecule).
Stimulation of secretion: Lipids in intestinal lumen, GRP
Inhibition of secretion: Somatostatin
Actions: Inhibits gastric secretion, stimulates pancreatic exocrine secretion (to take fatty acids up), stimulates motility of colon and small intestine, trophic factor for colon mucosa (possible relevance in colon cancer). [33, 41]

Peptide YY (PYY)

Localisation and production: PYY is a member of the pancreatic polypeptide family together with pancreatic polypeptide (PP) and neuropeptide Y (NPY). It is produced in endocrine cells of the ileum, colon and rectum.
Structure: There are two different forms: PYY 1-36 and PYY3-36.
Stimulation of secretion: Luminal contents, especially fat directly (open-type cells) or indirectly via GRP and CCK, vagal-stimulation
Inhibition of secretion: unknown
Actions: Slows down intestinal motility, inhibits gastric secretion and emptying, small intestine motility and pancreatic enzyme secretion. Perhaps relevant for satiety (high levels lead supress hunger; low levels stimulate hunger). [33, 41, 42, 51]

Pancreatic Polypeptide (PP)

Localisation and production: PP is produced in the PP-cells in the periphery of pancreatic islets.
Structure: It consists of 36 amino-acids.
Stimulation of secretion: Gastric distension, hypoglycaemia, vagal stimulation, nutrients
Inhibition of secretion: somatostatin, hyperglycemia, GRP
Actions: Inhibits pancreatic exocrine secretion, reducing gastric emptying and upper intestinal motility, inducing satiety. [33, 41, 42]

Ghrelin

Localisation and production: It is produced in P/D1-cells that are found mainly in the stomach and to a lesser extent in the small and large intestine. Ghrelin is also synthesized in pancreatic A-cells.
Structure: Ghrelin is 28-amino-acid peptide, with structural similarities to motilin.
Stimulation of release: Fasting, stimulating gastric contraction
Inhibition of secretion: unknown
Actions: Stimulates appetite, regulates insulin sensitivity and hepatic glucose output, cardiovascular effects (vasodilation, improvement of left ventricular contractility), stimulates growth hormone secretagogue receptor (GHS-R) and thereby stimulates growth. [33, 41]

Chromogranin-A related proteins

Through various proteolytic steps, members of the Chromogranin-family can be transformed into bioactive peptides. Examples are pancreastatin, which is known to inhibit insulin release and increase plasma glucose by activating hepatic glycogenolysis. Further examples are vasostatin 1 and 2, parastatin or secretoneurin. These substances are thought to act both pro- and anti-inflammatory. [33, 37, 41, 43]

Peptides acting predominantly on neurones (neurotransmitter)

Vasoactive intestinal polypeptide (VIP)

Localisation: It belongs to a family of proteins also including PACAP, peptide histidine methionine (PHM) and peptide histamine isoleucin (PHI), which are all neurotransmitters and found in various locations in the CNS, PNS and gastrointestinal tract.
Structure: VIP is a 28 AA polypeptide
Actions: Released by duodenal acidification and gastric distension. Relaxes lower oesophageal sphincter, Sphincter Oddi, Pylorus, modifies gut motility (contracts longitudinal and relaxes circular muscle in small intestine) and blood circulation, Stimulates bicarbonate secretion (duodenal glands, pancreas, liver), inhibits gastric secretion [33, 41]

Pituitary Adenylate Cyclase-Activating Peptide (PACAP)

Localisation: Found from the esophagus to the colon
Structure: There are two forms of PACAP in the gastrointestinal tract - PACAP 38 and PACAP 27. Via three receptors (PAC1, VPAC1, VPAC2) it increases intracellular cAMP in CNS and PNS.
Actions: Stimulates histamine release from stomach, secretion of exocrine pancreas, insulin and catecholamins. [33, 41]

Gastrin-releasing peptide (GRP) and Bombesin-like family of peptides

Localisation: GRP can be found in CNS, PNS, nerves of the gastrointestinal tract, the lungs and the genitourinary systems.
Structure: Bombesin was first isolated from amphibians and was then shown to be present in humans as GRP. It is related to neuromedin B and neuromedin C (both decapeptides) and consists of 27 aminoacids.

Actions: Stimulates contraction of stomach, intestine and gallbladder. Stimulates release of CCK, gastrin, GIP, glucacon, GLP-1, GLP-2, motilin, PP, PYY, somatostatin. Growth factor for cells in lung, pancreas. Perhaps promotes endocrine neoplasms in lung, pancreas. Neuromedin B also inhibits thyreotropin release. [33, 41, 52]

Calcitonin gene-related peptide (CGRP)

Localisaiton: Found mainly in cells in the small intestine and rectum
Structure: CGRP is a 37 amino-acid peptide, which is transcribed from the same gene as calcitonin (CALC-A, CALC-B) but is modified by alternative splicing of RNA. There are two forms: α-CGRP and β-CRGP, the latter being predominant in enteric neurons.
Actions: Released upon intraluminal glucose and acid secretion in the stomach, causes vasodilation in GI-tract, inhibiting gastric acid and pancreatic secretion. [33, 41]

Tachykinins

Substance P, neurokinin A and neurokinin B belong to the tachykinins

Localisation: Found in the CNS and PNS, the lungs, skin, sensory organs, urogenital tract and in EC cells.
Structure: Substance P: 11-amino acid peptide; all tachykinins share a C-terminal sequence
Actions: Vasodilatation, vasoconstriction, effects intestinal smooth muscles. [33, 41]

Neuropeptide Y (NPY)

Localisation: It is produced in CNS and PNS but also in the pancreatic islets.
Structure: NPY is a 36 aminoacid peptide related to PYY and PP.
Actions: Vasoconstriction, antisecretory effects, inhibits insulin secretion. [33, 41]

Galanin

Localisation: Galanin is found in CNS, PNS, pancreas, liver and in myenteric and submucosal plexus in the gut, lung and urogential tract.

Structure: Two different human forms of galanin exist: Galanin 19 (amino acids) and Galanin 30.

Actions: Regulates food intake, emomy and cognition, antinociception, inhibits pancreatic exocrine secretion, delayin gastric emptying and prolongs colonic transit times. [33, 41]

Thyrotropin-releasing hormone (TRH)

Localisation: TRH is not only produced in the hypothalamus but also in in the GI-tract (stomach, colon, pancreas). It is produced in pancreatic β-cells, G cells in the stomach and in neurons.

Structure: Consists of 3 amino acids.

Actions: Modulates pancreatic blood flow, gastric mucosal permeability, suppresses gastric acid secretion. [33, 41]

3.4 Molecular basics of neuroendocrine tumorigenesis

The molecular mechanisms leading to oncogenesis of neuroendocrine cells are only elucidated to a small extent. Although new techniques of analysing genetic alterations provide new insights into some of the underlying mechanisms, the results achieved so far are only fragmental.

The most important methods in analysing gene mutations and gene expression patterns are (cf. [53, 54]):

- Comparative genomic hybridization (CGH), which enables the investigator to visualise gains and losses in chromosomes; [53, 54]

- Loss of heterozygosity (LOH) – analysis: A patient may inherit a mutated allele of a gene from one parental side – the patient then is heterozygous for this mutation. In the process of oncogenesis the corresponding wild-type (normal, "healthy") allele is mutated too, leading to a homozygous mutation (loss of heterozygosity). This is an important process both for inactivation of tumour-suppressor genes and activation of tumour-promoting genes. [53, 54]
- DNA microarray chip - gene expression analysis: This technique can be used both for visualisation of distinct DNA mutations (also small losses and amplifications) or for quantitative and qualitative detection of RNA, that corresponds with the production of the protein, for which a gene encodes. [53, 54]

Pancreatic neuroendocrine tumours have been investigated more accurately than other gastrointestinal neuroendocrine tumours. For both it has been shown that mutations of tumour suppressor- and oncogenes involved in malignant transformation of gastrointestinal adenocarcinoma (e.g. K-Ras, p53, DCC, PTEN) are rarely found. [53, 54]

The underlying defects in familial tumour-syndromes associated with gastrointestinal neuroendocrine tumours (MEN1, Von-Hippel-Lindau [VHL]) have been well elucidated and are known to be relevant in sporadic neuroendocrine tumour disease too. For example, the mutation in the Menin-gene (located on chromosome 11q13) found in MEN1 leads to a defect Menin-protein. Menin normally inhibits JunD (a transcription factor) mediated cell proliferation. If the Menin-gene is defective, the JunD-mechanism is "out of control". A LOH-mutation on chromosome 11q13 is found in 80% of MEN1-associated tumours, but only in 21% of sporadic pancreatic NETs (8% insulinoma, 37% gastrinoma, 44% Vipoma, 67% glucagonoma). [53, 54]

In the VHL-syndrome, the VHL-gene (on chromosome 3p25-26) is mutated. The VHL-gene is a tumour-suppressor gene degrading hypoxia-inducible factor (HIF), a transcription factor that induces cell proliferation. A mutation in VHL-gene is found in most pancreatic NETs in patients suffering from VHL whereas it is hardly detected in sporadic tumours. However 33% of pancreatic NETs show LOH mutations on the 3p chromosome which is very likely important due to other tumour-suppressor genes located there (not known so far). [53, 54]

Recent studies compare genetic mutations and gene expression in metastatic pancreatic neuroendocrine tumours with non-metastasized tumours and with normal pancreatic islet cells. These analyses show the correlation of quantity of genetic alterations (chromosomal losses and gains; over-/underexpression of genes) with grade of malignancy (the more genetic differences, the higher the grade of malignancy). Genes, that were overexpressed in pancreatic NETs were either known to be putative oncogenes or encoding for growth factors or associated proteins such as insulin-like-growth-factor-binding-protein 3 (IGFBP3; which prolongs the half-life-time of IGF), cell adhesion and migration proteins, proteins associated with angiogenesis, remodelling, signal-transduction and Ca-dependent cell signalling. Underexpressed genes encoded for cell cycle check proteins and proteins for DNA damage repair and genomic stability. [53, 54]

Another interesting detail observed by Carpuso et al is the analogy of genetic defects in primary tumour and metastases. The author hypothesizes that this is due to the fact that neuroendocrine tumours develop a metastatic potential at a very early stage in transformation which leads to early metastatic disease even in small primary tumours. [55]

CGH revealed gains (most frequent 5q, 12q, 18q, 20q) and losses (most frequent 3p, 6pq, 10pq) at many chromosomes in pancreatic NETs suggesting that these are locations for other tumour suppressor/promotor genes unknown so far. [53, 54]

Gastrointestinal NETs at locations other than the pancreas have been under far less investigation. It is known so far that the molecular profiles of bronchial, pancreatic and other gastrointestinal NETs differ clearly. One study showed that the number of mutations is smaller than in pancreatic NETs and that there is no clear correlation of quantity of changes and grade of malignancy, as observed in pancreatic NETs. [56]

A high proportion of loss of the entire chromosome 18 was reported in GI-NETs (up to 84% [57]).

In summary, there are many unanswered questions regarding the mechanisms of neuroendocrine oncogenesis. The variability of symptoms and the differences in biological behaviour of gastrointestinal neuroendocrine tumours suggest big differences in the genetics of this tumour entity. [53, 54]

4. Neuroendocrine tumours of the gastrointestinal tract

4.1 Histopathological findings

4.1.1 Morphology and microscopy

Histomorphological findings in gastrointestinal neuroendocrine tumour disease are described as follows:

"... In the appendix they appear as bulbous swellings of the tip, which frequently obliterate the lumen. Elsewhere in the gut, they appear as intramural or submucosal masses that create small, polypoid, or plateau-like elevations rarely more than 3 cm in diameter. The overlying mucosa may be intact or ulcerated, and the tumors may permeate the bowel wall to invade the mesentery. A characteristic feature is a solid, yellow-tan appearance on transection. The tumors are exceedingly firm owing to striking desmoplasia, and when these fibrosing lesions penetrate the mesentery of the small bowel, they may cause angulation of kinking sufficient to result in obstruction. When present, visceral metastases are usually small, dispersed nodules and rarely reach the size seen with primary lesions.

Histologically the neoplastic cells may form discrete islands, trabeculae, glands, or undifferentiated sheets. Whatever their organization, the tumor cells are monotonously similar, having a scant, pink, granular cytoplasm and a round-to-oval stippled nucleus. In most tumors, there is minimal variation in cell and nuclear size, and mitoses are infrequent or absent. In unusual cases, there may be more significant anaplasia and sometimes mucin secretion within the cells and gland formations. Rarely tumors arise resembling small cell carcinomas of the lung or contain abundant psammoma bodies similar to those seen in papillary thyroid carcinomas. By electron microscopy, the cells in most tumors contain cytoplasmic, membrane-bound secretory granules with osmiophilic centers (dense-core granules). Most carcinoids can be shown to contain chromogranin A, synaptophysin and neuron-specific enolase." [58]

4.1.2 Immunohistochemistry

Although former diagnosis was only based on microscopical findings, nowadays immunohistochemistry is mandatory – only the combination of both techniques can make the diagnosis "neuroendocrine tumour" sure.

In general, every marker of neuroendocrine differentiation, including cytosolic, synaptic and cell adhesion molecules, can be used. However, chromogranin A and synaptophysin are thought to be especially important and invaluable [35, 59-61] and both the WHO classification [62, 63] and the recent "Guidelines for the Diagnosis and Treatment of Neuroendocrine Gastrointestinal Tumours" published by the European Neuroendocrine Tumour Society [64] are based upon histopathological diagnosis with these two markers. The combination of (at least) two or three neuroendocrine markers is thought to be the optimal approach since with de-differentiation cells may lose their ability to express LDCVs and thus are in turn negative for chromogranin A [35] (as some somatostatin-producing cells are too). Additionally, there are also cell types with low expression of synaptophysin [34]. Chromogranin A, synaptophysin, NSE and PGP9.5 are used most often in everyday routine – however, the first two should be performed in any case and contained in any combination of neuroendocrine markers. It is worth noting that the use of NSE has certain limitations because of its unspecific reactions to various closely related isoforms [62].

Immunohistochemistry can also be used for assessing cell proliferation (especially Ki-67 index; a marker showing quantity of mitoses by detection of the Ki-67-protein that is only present in G1, S, G2 and M phase in cell cycle [but not in G0] with a monoclonal antibody [MIB-1]). Nonetheless, reliable markers for the prediction of biological behaviour, speed of growth and potential to metastasize are absent for neuroendocrine tumour disease [61].

Immunohistochemistry (just like autoradiography [especially in frozen tissue]) is furthermore used for detecting specific peptide receptors on (GEP) neuroendocrine tumours. Somatostatin receptors, mostly sst2, are expressed most often in GEP-NETs (and to a higher amount than in "healthy" neuroendocrine tissue) but also GLP-1, CCK-2 (both highly in insulinomas), VIP-, Bombesin-, NPY- and Secretin-receptors. Quantitative (receptor density) and qualitative (receptor subtypes) detection of receptors is important for developing both diagnostic and therapeutic strategies (especially somatostatin-receptors) [65].

Staining techniques for specific hormones can also be applied for detecting a specific cell type of the tumour's origin. For pancreatic, duodenal and small intestine NETs especially, the detection of hormones in the tumour in relation to clinical syndrome is of interest.

4.2 Classification

4.2.1 Former nomenclature and classifications

Since S. Oberndorfer coined the term "Karzinoid" in 1907, the nomenclature and classification of neuroendocrine tumours has caused quite a bit of confusion. The term carcinoid was used for any tumour of gastrointestinal endocrine cells independent of its biological activity (hormone production), behaviour, differentiation and localisation.

Williams and Sandler (original work [66]) were the first to publish a classification for neuroendocrine tumours by subdividing them according to embryologic criteria into foregut (lung, stomach, duodenum, pancreas, upper jejunum), midgut (lower jejunum, ileum, appendix and cecum) and hindgut (colon and rectum) carcinoids. This concept, although sometimes still in use, did not turned out to be useful: Tumours of different localisations in one group (e.g. lung and pancreas in foregut carcinoids) differ extremely and should not be put in the category. In 1980 the WHO first tried to reclassify neuroendocrine tumours still using the term carcinoid for any tumour. With the growing knowledge about this very special tumour entity and international consensus conferences, the WHO revised its classification and published a recent one in 2000. [62, 63, 67]

4.2.2 WHO Classification 2000

The WHO classification published in 2000[63] uses the neutral and more general term "neuroendocrine tumour" for defining tumours of endocrine origin. It is based upon the assumption that all neuroendocrine tumours are potentially malignant but have a different biological behaviour (capacity to metastasize). Thus, tumours are subdivided into neuroendocrine tumours and neuroendocrine carcinomas. The term "carcinoid" was limited to neuroendocrine tumours, which can either be benign or of uncertain malignant potential. Neuroendocrine carcinomas (the term "malignant carcinoid" is valid for this group) are malignant by definition and can further be subdivided into well-differentiated neuroendocrine carcinomas (with low-grade malignancy) and poorly-differentiated neuroendocrine carcinomas (usually small cell, with high-grade malignancy). This tumour classification is applied to any localisation in the gastrointestinal tract (stomach, duodenum + proximal jejunum, ileum + distal jejunum, appendix, colon-rectum and pancreas; in practical terms the whole jejunum is often combined with the ileum; and colon and rectum NETs are split up). The WHO classification additionally includes mixed exocrine-endocrine tumours (either with exocrine or endocrine cells as leading component; endocrine component at least 1/3 or ½ of tumour cells) and for pancreatic tumours, also tumour-like lesions (see **Table 2**). (cf. [62, 63])

WHO-Group 1	(a) Well-differentiated neuroendocrine tumour benign (b) Uncertain malignant potential
WHO-Group 2	Well-differentiated neuroendocrine carcinoma malignant
WHO-Group 3	Poorly differentiated neuroendocrine carcinoma malignant
Additional (WHO-Group 4)	Mixed exocrine-endocrine carcinoma malignant
Additional (WHO-Group 5)	Tumorlike lesions (only in pancreatic NETs) benign

Table 2 - Classification of neuroendocrine tumors of the gastroenteropancreatic system (GEP-NET); adapted after [62]

The differentiation into benign, uncertain and malignant tumours is based upon various criteria (see **Table 3** and **Table 4**): Firstly, tumour size is important for estimating a neuroendocrine tumour's behaviour. Tumour size smaller than 2cm for pancreatic NETs and size smaller than 1cm for intestinal NETs is associated with a close to 100% probability of benign behaviour. Further important criteria are angioinvasion, histological differentiation and Ki-67 index, invasion of adjacent organs (in pancreatic NETs) or the muscularis propria layer (in intestinal NETs), hormonal activity and presence of specific hormonal syndromes. [62, 63]

Biological behaviour	Tumour size (cm)	Invasion of muscularis propria	Histological differentiation	Angio-invasion	Ki-67 index (%)	Hormonal syndrome	Metastases
Benign	≤1 [a]	-	Well differentiated	-	<2	- [a]	-
Benign or low-grade	≤2	-	Well differentiated	-/+	<2	-	-
Low-grade malignant	>2	+ [b]	Well differentiated	+	>2	+	+
High-grade malignant	Any	+	Poorly differentiated	+	>20	+	+

[a] Exception: malignant duodenal gastrinomas are usually smaller than 1cm and confined to the submucosa
[b] Exception: benign NETs of the appendix usually invade the muscularis propria

Table 3 - Criteria for assessing the prognosis of neuroendocrine tumours of the intestine [62, 63]

Biological behaviour	Tumour size (cm)	Invasion of muscularis propria	Histological differentiation	Angio-invasion	Ki-67 index (%)	Hormonal syndrome	Metastases
Benign	≤1	-	Well differentiated	-	<2	- [a]	-/+ [b]
Benign or low-grade	>2	-	Well differentiated	-/+	<2	-	-/+ [c]
Low-grade malignant	>3	+	Well differentiated	+	>2	+	+ [c]
High-grade malignant	Any	+	Poorly differentiated	+	>20	+	-

[a] Invasion of adjacent organs (e.g. duodenum, stomach)
[b] Insulinomas
[c] Insulinomas and other functioning tumours (e.g. glucagonomas)

Table 4 - Criteria for assessing the prognosis of neuroendocrine tumours of the pancreas [62, 63]

Although the new classification has brought much improvement to unifying the diagnosis and classification of GEP-NETs, there are various critical points about it: Firstly, the definition "uncertain malignant potential" is unsatisfactory . A grading system should imply sufficient information about the prognosis of a tumour disease. Additionally, although several studies showed a significant correlation between Ki-67 index and progression of neuroendocrine tumour disease (for review see [68]), assessment of Ki-67 index has certain limitations: The cut-off levels (<2, >2, >20) are still under discussion and a correct diagnosis depends on (and may vary with) both the experience of the pathologist and the availability of adequate material (biopsy may only represent a part of a tumour).

4.2.3 WHO Classification 2010

Because of a low rate of acceptance in the USA and the fact that grading and staging criteria where merged within the WHO 2000 classification, in 2010 the WHO developed a revised version of its classification for neuroendocrine tumours[69]. The new system now consists of a grading system (G1, G2, G3) that is combined with a site-specific staging-system (identical with the AJCC/UICC-TNM-System).
The terms "benign" tumor and "tumor of uncertain clinical behaviour" now do not exist anymore. A tumour is now determinated by its grading and staging using the TNM-System. [69]
In the **Table 5** the new definition of the WHO-groups is given. The grading is in accordance to the one developed by ENETS (see 4.2.4) whereas the TNM-staging equals the AJCC/UICC system (see 4.2.5).

WHO-Group	WHO 2000	WHO 2010
1	Well-differentiated endocrine tumour (benign or uncertain)	Neuroendorine Tumour (NET) G1 (carcinoid)
2	Well-differentiated endocrine carcinoma	Neuroendocrine Tumour (NET) G2
3	Poorly differentiated endocrine carcinoma/smal cell carcinoma	Neuroendocrine Carcinoma (NEC) G3
4	Mixed exocrine-endocrine carcinoma	Mixed adenoneuroendocrine carcinoma (MANEC)
5	Tumour-like lesions (TLL)	Hyperplastic and preoplastic lesions

G1: mitotic count <2 per 10 high power fields (HPF) and/or ≤2% Ki67 index
G2: mitotic count 2-20 per 10 HPF and/or 3-20%Ki67 index
G3: mitotic count >20 per 10 HPF and/or20% Ki67 index

Table 5 - Comparison of the WHO 2000 and the WHO 2010 classification of neuroendocrine neoplasms of the digestive system (after [69])

4.2.4 European Neuroendocrine Tumor Society (ENETS) Grading and TNM Classification

For staging of disease both a grading and a TNM-classification comparable to other carcinomas have been proposed in 2006 and 2007 by the European Neuroendocrine Tumor Society [70, 71].

A tumour's grade is assessed by either mitotic count or Ki-67 index (see **Table 6**).

The pTNM-classifications for each localisation are given in chapter 4.3.

Grade	Mitotic count (10HPF[a])	Ki-67 index (%[b])
G1	<2	≤2
G2	2-20	3-20
G3	>20	>20

[a]Ten HPF: high power field=2mm², at least 40 fields evaluated in areas at highest mitotic density
[b]MiB1 antibody; Percent of 2000 cells in areas of highest nuclear labelling

Table 6 - Proposal for a grading system for neuroendocrine tumours [70, 71]

4.2.5 AJCC/UICC TNM-classificiation

In 2009 the American Joint Cancer Committee (AJCC) and the Union Internationale Contre le Cancer (UICC) published their 7th edition of the "TNM classification of malignant tumour"[72]. 3 years after the publication of the ENETS TNM system, these societies, which mainly influence Northern American oncologic centers, presented their proposal for the grading and staging of gastrointestinal neuroendocrine tumours. Although the two systems are concordant in most points, some differences in the T-classification and staging of tumours in the stomach, the appendix and the pancreas exist. Especially the differences in the T-classification and staging for pancreatic and appendiceal tumours were critisised [73].

Because the clinical relevance of the ENETS TNM-system is already evident [74, 75] and the parallel existence of two TNM-systems is confusing, in the following only the ENETs TNM system is used.

However, the detailed information for the AJCC/UICC T-classification for every site is given in chapter 4.3 next to the ENETS-T-classification.

4.2.6 Mixed neuroendocrine/non-neuroendocrine tumours

On the one hand mixed neuroendocrine/exocrine tumours can contain neuroendocrine and non-neuroendocrine signs either as clearly distinguishable parts (one part of the tumour consiting of neuroendocrine cells; the other part of non-neuroendocrine cells). On the other hand these tumours can consist of cells, that contain both qualities. The first tumours are called mixed neuroendocrine/exocrine tumours, the latter are termed "goblet-cell-carcinoma". Goblet-cell carincomas consist of tumour cells expressing both neuroendocrine granules but also exocrine products (so called amphicrine cells). [76]

Focal neuroendocrine differentiation is found in many non-neuroendocrine tumours (in the GI-tract but also lung and breast). As mentioned above a tumour should only be called mixed neuroendocrine/exocrine tumour if the neuroendocrine compartment exceeds at least 30% of all tumour cells. [76]

4.3 Specific findings at each localisation

4.3.1 Neuroendocrine tumours of the oesophagus

Pathological findings

Oesophageal neuroendocrine tumours are rare neuroendocrine tumours. Most often they present as poorly differentiated neuroendocrine carcinomas (WHO-Group 3) and mixed endocrine-exocrine carcinomas. There are also rare cases of well-differentiated neuroendocrine tumours (WHO-Group 1 and 2). [77]

There is no accepted grading and staging-system for NETs of the oesophagus.

Clinical findings

Poorly differentiated NETs are found most often when already metastasized to lymph nodes or infiltrating adjacent organs. Their clinical presentation is therefore similar to oesophageal adeno- or squamous-cell carcinomas. They have a poor prognosis. Only rare cases of associated paraneoplastic syndromes were reported (Ectopic production of ADH and VIP).

Well-differentiated NETs of the oesophagus show far better long-term prognosis and lymph-node metastases are not normally found. [77]

4.3.2 Neuroendocrine tumours of the stomach

Pathological findings

NETs of the stomach, especially the well-differentiated ones, most often arise from ECL cells, although there are also rare cases of tumours deriving from G-cells, D-cells or EC-cells. ECL-cells highly express VMAT2, which is used to detect these cells especially. Although in incidence studies these tumours are rather rare, some authors consider these tumours to be the most frequent NETs in the digestive system [62].

Gastric NETs can be subdivided into three fundamental subgroups (or four subgroups when including poorly-differentiated tumours) (cf. [80])

Gastric NET Type 1 (WHO-Group 1): These are the most frequent gastric NETs, associated with chronic atrophic gastritis (CAG) and localised in the corpus of the stomach. Women are affected more frequently. The tumours are often polypoid and multiple, having a diameter of about 0,5 to 1cm. They consist of ECL cells (producing histamine). In CAG, the acid-producing parietal-cells of the stomach are destroyed. As a consequence, G-cells overproduce gastrin, which aims to stimulate acid production. This results in an overstimulation of ECL-cells and ECL hyperplasia and further in the formation of multiple neuroendocrine tumours. However hypergastrinemia is most likely only a side effect since overexpression of other growth factors (e.g. TGF-α) can be detected in these tumours. [78]

Gastric NET Type 2: These are caused by primary hypergastrinemia in Zollinger-Ellison-Syndrome (see below) are very rare and only in patients suffering from MEN1-syndrome. The NETs are also multiple, localised in the corpus and combined with ECL-cell hyperplasia but they are localised in a hyperplastic mucosa and are mainly benign (WHO-group 1). There is no tendency towards a higher affliction in females. These tumours rarely metastasize when exceeding 1-2cm of size or when angioinvasion is present (WHO-group 2). [78]

Gastric NET Type 3 (WHO-group 2): These are sporadic tumours and most often solitary. They consist most often of ECL-cells, seldom of G-cells or EC-cells and are usually localised in the fundus/gastric corpus and sometimes also in the antrum. They are predominantly found in male patients and in 1/3 of the patients larger than 2cm at time of diagnosis, with a Ki-67 >2% and evidence of infiltration of the muscularis propria. If this is the case, locoregional lymph node metastases are frequent. [78]

Poorly differentiated neuroendocrine carcinomas (Gastric NET Type 4; WHO-group 3): These carcinomas were also called small-cell carcinomas or oat-cell carcinoma. The staining for synaptophysin is positive whereas chromogranin A is only poorly expressed or negative. They are detected at an advanced stage (larger than 4cm). [79]

Mixed exocrine-endocrine carcinomas in the stomach should be generally counted and treated as adenocarcinomas. [77]

Clinical findings

Gastric NETs Type 1, especially, may produce hardly any symptoms and are diagnosed incidentally during gastroscopy for either dyspepsia or macrocytic anemia, most often at in patients approximately 50-70 years of age. Poorly differentiated neuroendocrine carcinomas are clinically similar to adenocarcinomas and cause pain, bleeding or obstruction with a bad prognosis (causing death within 1 year in 75% of patients). [64, 77-79]

Atypical carcinoid syndrome from gastric NETs Type 3 is very rare and characterized by flush, diarrhoea, swelling and asthma due to histamine overproduction. Gastrin overproduction (gastrinoma) from gastric NETs Type 3 have been described but are extremely rare. [64, 77-79] Up to 50% of the patients suffering from NETs Type 3 die due to the tumour. [79]

WHO	
1	**Well-differentiated neuroendocrine tumour (carcinoid)** Benign: non-functioning, confined to mucosa-submucosa, nonangioinvasive, ≤1cm in size • ECL cell tumour of corpus-fundus (usually multiple) associated with chronic atrophic gastritis (CAG) or MEN-1 syndrome • Serotonin-producing or (very rare) gastrin-producing tumour Benign or low grade malignant (uncertain malignant potential): non-functioning, confined to mucosa-submucosa, with or without angioinvasion, >1-2cm in size • ECL cell tumor with CAG or MEN-1 syndrome or sporadic • Serotonin-producing or (very rare) gastrin-producing tumour
2	**Well-differentiated neuroendocrine carcinoma (malignant carcinoid)** Low grade malignant: invasion of the muscularis propria and beyond or metastases; >2cm in size • Nonfunctioning: usally sporadic ECL cell carcinoma, rarely in CAG/MEN-1 or serotonin or gastrin-producing • Functioning with serotonin-producing carcinoma (atypical carcinoid syndrome) or gastrin-producing carcinoma (gastrinoma)
3	**Poorly differentiated neuroendocrine carcinoma** High grade malignant

Table 7 - Overview about the classification of neuroendocrine tumours of the stomach; taken from [62]

Abbreviation	Characteristics	
T - primary tumour; For any T add (m) for multiple tumours	ENETS	AJCC/UICC
TX	Primary tumour cannot be assessed	Primary tumour cannot be assessed
T0	No evidence of primary tumour	No evidence of primary tumour
Tis	In situ tumour/dysplasia (<0,5cm)	In situ tumour/dysplasia (<0,5cm)
T1	Tumour invades lamina propria or submcuosa and ≤ 1cm	Tumour confined to mucosa and 0.5mm or more but ≤ 1cm in size; or invades submucosa and ≤ 1cm in size
T2	Tumour invades muscularis propria or subserosa or > 1cm	Tumour invades muscularis propria or is > 1cm in size
T3	Tumour penetrates serosa	Tumour invades subserosa
T4	Tumour invades adjacent structures	Tumour perforates visceral peritoneum or other organs or adjacent structures
N – regional lymph nodes		
NX	Regional lymph node status cannot be assessed	
N0	No regional lymph node metastases	
N1	Regional lymph node metastases	
M – distant metastases		
MX	Distant metastases cannot be assessed	
M0	No distant metastases	
M1	Distant metastases	

Table 8 - Proposal for a pTNM classification for neuroendocrine tumours of the stomach; taken from [70, 72]

Stage	T	N	M
Stage 0	Tis	N0	M0
Stage 1	T1	N0	M0
Stage 2a	T2	N0	M0
Stage 2b	T3	N0	M0
Stage 3a	T4	N0	M0
Stage 3b	Any T	N1	M0
Stage 4	Any T	Any N	M1

Table 9 - Proposal for disease staging for neuroendocrine tumours of the stomach; taken from [77]

4.3.3 Neuroendocrine tumours of the duodenum

Pathological findings

Duodenal NETs are rare among neuroendocrine tumours (1-4%). They are found in up to 90% of tumours in the first and second part of the duodenum. These are usually small (<2cm), polypoid, solitary tumours within the submucosa. Multiple tumours are often associated with MEN 1 – syndrome. [80]

Most often, duodenal NETs are gastrin-producing or gastrin-secreting (gastrinoma), followed by tumours producing somatostatin, serotonin or calcitonin (non-functional, well-differentiated tumous). Poorly differentiated carcinomas and gangliocytic paragangliomas can also be found in rare cases. [64, 79, 80]

Gastrinoma: These are well-differentiated tumours, showing gastrin-expression, localised ~75% in the duodenum and ~25% in the pancreas (70-85% of gastrinomas in total are localised in the proximal duodenum or pancreatic head, the so-called "gastrinoma triangle") that cause Zollinger-Ellison syndrome (ZES; clinical considerations see below) due to overproduction of gastrin. In MEN 1 – syndrome (20-30% of the cases), they are found as multiple tumours whereas sporadic tumours are usually solitary[81]. In up to 80%, regional lymph node metastases are present at time of diagnosis, and may even be sometimes larger than the primary tumours, leading to the false diagnosis of a pancreatic gastrinoma, for example (when metastasis is localised around the head of the pancreas)[77]. Liver metastases are seldom (10%). The prognosis (10-year survival) of well-differentiated gastrinomas is up to 90% [81].

Non-functioning duodenal NETs: Duodenal NETs may also produce gastrin without causing ZES. Some of the duodenal NETs also produce somatostatin, calcitonin and extremely rarely, insulin, glucagon or ACTH (clinical symptoms due to hormone-secretion being even more rare). Tumours with expression of somatostatin are usually located in the ampullary region and histologically contain psammoma bodies and stain only for synaptophysin (but not chromogranin A) – they are often associated with Neurofibromatosis von Recklinghausen. The prognosis of well-differentiated carcinoma is good (5-year survival of 80-85%). [80]

Gangliocytic paraganglioma: These are tumours consisting of three differentiated cell types: Endocrine cells, neural spindle cells and ganglionic cells. They are usually localised in the periampullary region. Often they are large (1,5 to 7cm) and infiltrating; nonetheless lymph node metastases are rare. [77]

Poorly differentiated neuroendocrine carcinoma (WHO-group 3): Normally they grow around the papilla of Vater, showing ulcerated tumours, sized about 2 to 3cm. They rarely express chromogranin A but stain for synaptophysin. At time of diagnosis, they usually present with lymph node and liver metastases, and result in a bad prognosis. [77]

Clinical findings

Gastrinomas/Zollinger-Ellison Syndrom (ZES): Due to a gastrin secreting tumour, the parietal cells of the stomach produce gastric acid excessively, causing severe peptic ulcera (sometimes recurrent) and gastroesophageal reflux disease. Most gastrinomas causing ZES are found in the duodenum, and about 25% in the pancreas[77]. Fasting gastrin levels are elevated, such as basal gastric acid production (gastric hypersecretion). The mean age of patients is about 48 to 55 years[81].

Others: 90% of duodenal NETs do not cause clinical syndrome. Major symptoms are thus pain, jaundice, nausea/vomiting, bleeding, anemia, diarrhea and obstruction. Syndromes other than ZES (Carcinoid-syndrome, Cushing's syndrome, acromegaly, somatostinoma syndrome, insulinoma, glucagonoma) are very rare. [80]

WHO	
1	**Well-differentiated neuroendocrine tumour (carcinoid)** Benign: non-functioning, confined to mucosa-submucosa, non-angioinvasive, ≤1cm in size • Gastrin-producing tumor (upper part of the duodenum) • Serotonin-producing • Gangliocytic paraganglioma (any size and extension, periampullary) Benign or low grade malignant (uncertain malignant potential): non-functioning, confined to mucosa-submucosa, with or without angioinvasion, >1-2cm in size • Functioning gastrin-producing tumor (gastrinoma), sporadic or MEN-1 associated • Nonfunctioning somatostatin-producing tumour (ampullary region) with or without neurofibromatosis type 1 • Nonfunctioning serotonin-producing or (very rare) gastrin-producing tumour
2	**Well-differentiated neuroendocrine carcinoma (malignant carcinoid)** Low grade malignant: invasion of the muscularis propria and beyond or metastases • Functioning gastrin-producing carcinoma (gastrinoma), sporadic or MEN-1 associated • Nonfunctioning somatostatin-producing carcinoma (ampullary region) with or without neurofibromatosis type 1 • Nonfunctioning or functioning carcinoma (with carcinoid syndrome) • Malignant gangliocytic paraganglioma
3	**Poorly differentiated neuroendocrine carcinoma** High grade malignant

Table 10 - Overview about the classification of neuroendocrine tumours of the duodenum and upper jejunum; taken from [62]

Abbreviation	Characteristics	
T - primary tumour; For any T add (m) for multiple tumours	ENETS	AJCC/UICC
TX	Primary tumour cannot be assessed	Primary tumour cannot be assessed
T0	No evidence of primary tumour	No evidence of primary tumour
T1	Tumour invades lamina propria or submucosa and ≤ 1cm	Tumour invades lamina propria or submucosa and ≤ 1cm
T2	Tumour invades muscularis propria or > 1cm	Tumour invades muscularis propria or is > 1cm in size
T3	Tumour invades pancreas or retroperitoneum (for duodenum, ampulla and proximal jejunum) Tumour invades serosa (for lower jejunum and ileum)	Ampullary or duodenal tumour invades pancreas or retroperitoneum Jejunal or ileal tumour invades subserosa
T4	Tumour invades peritoneum or other organs	Tumour perforates visceral peritoneum (serosa) or other organs or adjacent structures
N – regional lymph nodes		
NX	Regional lymph node status cannot be assessed	
N0	No regional lymph node metastases	
N1	Regional lymph node metastases	
M – distant metastases		
MX	Distant metastases cannot be assessed	
M0	No distant metastases	
M1	Distant metastases	

Table 11 - Proposal for a pTNM classification for neuroendocrine tumours of the duodenum/ampulla/jejunum and ileum; adapted from [70, 72]

Stage	T	N	M
Stage 1	T1	N0	M0
Stage 2a	T2	N0	M0
Stage 2b	T3	N0	M0
Stage 3a	T4	N0	M0
Stage 3b	Any T	N1	M0
Stage 4	Any T	Any N	M1

Table 12 - Proposal for disease staging for neuroendocrine tumours of the duodenum/ampulla/jejunum and ileum; adapted from [77]

4.3.4 Neuroendocrine tumours of the pancreas (PNETs)

Neuroendocrine tumours of the pancreas are rare tumours that usually grow as solitary tumours and are most often well differentiated. Multiple tumours are often associated with familiary tumour syndromes such as MEN1 or von-Hippel-Lindau. [77]

PNETs are subdivided into functioning and non-functioning tumours, according to whether they cause clinical symptoms or not [77]. Most of the PNETs belong to the group of well-differentiated carcinomas (WHO-group 2) [82]. As an exception, insulinomas are more often benign (WHO-group 1) [83].

70-80% of PNETs are non-functioning tumours[82]. Among the functioning, insulinomas are most frequent, followed by gastrinomas. VIPomas, glucagonomas and other hormone-secreting pancreatic tumours are extremely rare [64, 84]. Poorly-differentiated carcinomas are also infrequent among PNETs [77].

The WHO-criteria (**Table 4**) is reliable for the assessment of biological behaviour of PNETS[77]. Another immunohistochemical marker, Cytokeratin 19 (CK19), was shown to be helpful for classifying the PNETs specifically [85].

Pathological findings

Functioning PNETs

Functioning PNETs often show expression for more than one hormone, although immunohistochemically, the hormone which causes the clinical symptoms is predominant. [77]

Insulinomas

They most often belong into the WHO-group 1 (well-differentiated neuroendocrine tumours = benign). Only 8.4% of insulinomas are malignant. These are usually solitary tumours, sized 0.5-2cm. Histologically, deposits of amyloid can often be found in these cells. Normally immunohistochemical reactivity for both chromogranin A and synaptophysin such as expression of insulin and pro-insulin can be shown. [77, 83]

Gastrinomas

Pancreatic gastrinomas are less frequent than duodenal ones. They more often present with liver metastases (30%), but only seldom metastasize to other organs. 10-year survival-time with metastases is about 40-50%. [77, 81]

Glucagonomas

This very rare tumour usually is about 3 to 7cm in diameter and most often localised in the pancreas' tail. It shows hormonal immunoreactivity for glucagon or proglucagon-derived peptides. Metastases are found in 60-70%, but the tumour grows slowly. [77]

VIPomas

They stain for VIP and peptide histidine methionine (PHM) and are usually localised in the tail of the pancreas. Metastases are already present predominantely at time of diagnosis. [77]

Somatostatinoms

Even though the somatostatinoma syndrome was described already in 1979, many authors doubt its existence. This very rare, somatostatin-expressing tumour should be a non-functioning PNET. In about 50%, the tumours are malignant and as in somatostatin-expressing duodenal NETs, psammoma bodies can be found. [77]

Other functioning PNETs

Tumours secreting ACTH, GHRH, calcitonin and serotonin are extremely rare and are diagnosed late, when liver metastases are already present. Thus patients suffering from these tumours have rather short survival rate. [77]

Non-functioning PNETs

These tumours are most often incidental findings with modern imaging techniques such as CT-scan or MRT. They often show immunoreactivity for various hormones (Glucagon, somatostatin, pancreatic polypeptid, ACTH, calcitonin, parathyroid hormone) and the expression of a hormone sometimes causes elevated serum-levels of the expressed hormone too. Nonetheless if no clinical symptom is present, these tumours should be classified as non-functioning tumours (not glucagonona, somatostinoma). They are most often positive for both chromogranin A and synaptophysin (again with the exception of somatostatin-producing tumours) and are well-differentiated neuroendocrine carcinomas (WHO-group 2). Since they are often detected late, the 5-year survival rate is only 30-63%. [77, 82]

Poorly-differentiated PNETs

They are predominantly localised in the head of the pancreas and most often infiltrate the surrounding tissues, having a high mitotic rate. At the time of diagnosis they measure about 4cm. The tumour-cells are either small and seldom very large. Male patients are affected more often. [79]

Clinical presentation

Insulinoma

Tumours larger than 1cm in size tend to be symptomatic but also smaller tumors can be symptomatic. Hypoglycemia due to oversecretion of insulin and proinsulin can lead to multiple possible symptoms, which can be subdivided into two groups: Neurological symptoms include loss of consciousness, ambiopia, confusion, aggressiveness and seizures. Counteraction of adrenergic nerves causes nausea, sweating, weakness, adephagia and palpitations. The symptom triad defined by Allen Whipple in the 1930s, Whipple's triad, is still valuable for determining if a patient's symptoms are caused by hypoglycemia. The triad consist of each of the hypoglycemic symptoms mentioned above, a plasma glucose level of ≤40mg/dl and the relief of all of the symptoms after administration of glucose. [77, 83, 86]

Nonetheless, for confirming the diagnosis of organic hyperinsulinism, it is necessary to measure serum parameters (insulin, proinsulin, C-peptide) during a standardized 72-hour fast. [77, 83, 86]

Gastrinoma

see duodenal NETs above.

Glucagonoma

The typical complex of symptoms caused by autonomic glucagon-overexpression includes weight loss, anemia, mild diabetes mellitus, depression, diarrhea and most typically, a skin disease called necrolytic migratory erythema consisting of and characterised by blisters and swelling (present in up to 80% of glucagonomas) especially in regions exposed to pressure (buttocks, perinealregion etc.). [77, 86]

VIPoma

The symptoms caused by autonomic secretion of VIP and PHM are summed up under the term Verner-Morrison-Syndrom, also called WDHA-syndrome. WDHA stands for watery diarrhea (up to 20 liters/day), hypokaliemia, hypochlorhydria and alkalosis, the latter three caused by the diarrhea. The subsequent exsiccosis can by life-threatening. [77, 86]

Somatostatinoma

Symptoms related to over-production of somatostatin, first described in 1979, were diabetes mellitus, cholecystolithiasis, steatorrhea, hypochlorhydria and anemia. [77, 86] However, it is still under discussion wheter these are caused by the hormone overproduction or only were *(...) unspecific manifestations of large malignant PETs that happened to produce somatostatin* [87].

Other-functioning PNETs

Ectopic hormone production of ACTH can lead to Cushing's disease, calcitonin to diarrhea, serotonin to carcinonid-symptoms (see below) and GHRH to acromegalia. [77, 86]

Non-functioning PNETs

The lack of symptoms is most often the reason for the late diagnosis of these tumours. Major symptoms include abdominal pain due to invasion of adjacent organs, weight loss, anorexia, nausea, intra-abdominal bleeding, jaundice or palpable tumour mass. Modern imaging technologies and their increasing availability may help to diagnose non-functioning PNETs earlier and more frequently. [77, 82]

WHO	
1	**Well-differentiated neuroendocrine tumour** Benign: confined to pancreas, <2cm in size, non-angioinvasive, ≤2 mitoses/HPF and ≤2% Ki-67-positive cells • Functioning: insulinoma • Nonfunctioning Benign or low grade malignant (uncertain malignant potential): confined to pancreas, ≥2cm in size, >2 mitoses/HPF, >% Ki-67-positive cells or angioinvasive • Functioning: gastrinoma, insulinoma, VIPoma, glucagonoma, somatostatinoma or ectopic hormonal syndrome • Nonfunctioning
2	**Well-differentiated neuroendocrine carcinoma** Low grade malignant: invasion of adjacent organs and/or metastases • Functioning: gastrinoma, insulinoma, glucagonoma, VIPoma, somatostatinoma or ectopic hormonal syndrome • Nonfunctioning
3	**Poorly differentiated neuroendocrine carcinoma** High grade malignant

Table 13 - Overview about the classification of neuroendocrine tumours of the pancreas; taken from [62]

Abbreviation	Characteristics	
T - primary tumour; For any T add (m) for multiple tumours	ENETS	AJCC/UICC
TX	Primary tumour cannot be assessed	Primary tumour cannot be assessed
T0	No evidence of primary tumour	No evidence of primary tumour
Tis		Carcinoma in situ
T1	Limited to the pancreas and size <2cm	Tumour limited to the pancreas, ≤ 2cm in greatest dimension
T2	Limited to the pancreas and size 2-4 cm	Tumour limited to the pancreas, > 2cm in greatest dimension
T3	Limited to the pancreas and size >4cm or invading duodenum or bile duct	Tumour extends beyond the pancreas
T4	Invading the wall of adjacent large vessels (celiac axis or superior mesenteric artery), stomach, spleen, colon, adrenal gland	Tumour involves coeliac axis or superior mesenteric artery
N – regional lymph nodes		
NX	Regional lymph node status cannot be assessed	
N0	No regional lymph node metastases	
N1	Regional lymph node metastases	
M – distant metastases		
MX	Distant metastases cannot be assessed	
M0	No distant metastases	
M1	Distant metastases	

Table 14 - Proposal for a pTNM classification for neuroendocrine tumours of the pancreas; taken from [71, 72]

Stage	T	N	M
Stage 1	T1	N0	M0
Stage 2a	T2	N0	M0
Stage 2b	T3	N0	M0
Stage 3a	T4	N0	M0
Stage 3b	Any T	N1	M0
Stage 4	Any T	Any N	M1

Table 15 - Proposal for disease staging by ENETS for neuroendocrine tumours of the pancreas; taken from [77]

Stage	T	N	M
Stage 0	Tis	N0	M0
Stage 1a	T1	N0	M0
Stage 1b	T2	N0	M0
Stage 2a	T3	N0	M0
Stage 2b	T1, T2, T3	N1	M0
Stage 3	T4	N0	M0
Stage 4	Any T	Any N	M1

Table 16 – Proposal for disease staging by AJCC/UICC for neuroendocrine tumours of the pancreas; taken from [72]

4.3.5 Neuroendocrine tumours of the jejunum, ileum and Meckel's diverticulum

According to literature neuroendocrine tumours of the small intestine (excluding the duodenum) are responsible for about 25% of all gastrointestinal neuroendocrine tumours. These are usually solitary tumours but in 26 to 30%, multicentric tumours can be found. Male and female patients are equally affected, most often between the 6th and 7th decade of life. Most of these NETs are well-differentiated carcinomas (WHO-group 2). [88]

Functioning and non-functioning tumours can be subdivided, although clinical symptoms due to hormone (serotonin) overproduction is found nearly exclusively in patients with liver-metastases (95%). [88]

The incidence of poorly-differentiated NETs in the small intestine is unknown – these are clearly extremely rare tumours, that histologically correlate to poorly-differentiated NETs of the colon and rectum (small- or large – cell carcinomas). [89]

Pathological findings

The tumours are usually more than 2cm in size (between 0.5 and 3cm). A size larger than 1cm is most often associated with infiltration of the muscularis propria and the subserosal fatty tissue. Lymph node metastases are found in 85% of tumours larger than 2cm. Lymph node metastases may be larger than the primary tumour. The tumour cells usually show the expression profile of an EC-cell (incl. pos. for serotonin) and are surrounded by a sclerotic stroma consisting of few cells. This stroma often causes kinking of the intestine, which results in obstruction and may be one of the first tumour associated symptoms. [77]

NETs in a Meckel's diverticulum are incidental findings and usually small (<1.7cm). [77]

Clinical findings

Overall 5-year survival is 50-60%. Presence of liver metastases diminishes the 5-year survival to 35%. [88]

Non-functioning tumours

They are usually found during surgical exploration due to newly diagnosed liver metastases or during colonoscopy in the distal ileum. If so, these tumours are larger than 2cm in size. Symptoms may not exceed abdominal discomfort; sometimes irritable bowel-syndrome is present for many years. As mentioned above tumour-fibrosis may lead to bowel obstruction or subileus. Later one fibrosis around lymph-node metastases can cause small bowel ischemia and hydronephrosis. [88]

Functioning tumours/Carcinoid syndrome

Without liver metastases it is very unlikely that an overproduction of serotonin causes symptoms – the liver degrades serotonin from the portal vein. If metastases are producing serotonin in the liver, then serotonin is released into the circulation and may produce typical syndromes including flush, diarrhoea, intermittent bronchoconstriction and later ‚carcinoid heart disease. Carcinoid crisis is defined as an acute exacerbation, often caused by anesthesia, invasive procedures incl. surgery as well as nutritional components. Bronchoconstriction, diarrhoea and cardiac arrhythmias can even be life-threatening. [88]

Carcinoid heart disease affects the right side of the heart, causing fibrosis of the tricuspid valve but also pulmonary valve with fixation and increasing insufficiency of the valves. Effects on the heart by a functioning neuroendocrine tumour with carcinoid-syndrome develop in 40-50% and may be responsible for death in up to 50%. [88]

1	**Well-differentiated neuroendocrine tumour (carcinoid)** Benign: non-functioning, confined to mucosa-submucosa, non-angioinvasive, ≤1cm (ileum) or ≤ 2cm (colon-rectum) • Serotonin-producing tumour • Enteroglucagon-producing tumour Benign or low grade malignant (uncertain malignant potential): non-functioning, confined to mucosa-submucosa, angioinvasive, >1cm (ileum) or >2cm (colon rectum) • Serotonin-producing tumour • Enteroglucagon-producing tumour
2	**Well-differentiated neuroendocrine carcinoma (malignant carcinoid)** Low grade malignant: invasion of the muscularis propria or beyond or metastases • Non-functioning or functioning serotonin-producing carcinoma (with carcinoid syndrome) • Non-functioning enteroglucagon-producing carcinoma
3	**Poorly differentiated neuroendocrine carcinoma** High grade malignant

Table 17 - Overview of the classification of neuroendocrine tumours of the ileum, cecum, colon and rectum; taken from [62]

Abbreviation	Characteristics	
T - primary tumour; For any T add (m) for multiple tumours	**ENETS**	**AJCC/UICC**
TX	Primary tumour cannot be assessed	Primary tumour cannot be assessed
T0	No evidence of primary tumour	No evidence of primary tumour
T1	Tumour invades lamina propria or submcuosa and ≤ 1cm	Tumour invades lamina propria, muscularis mucosae or submocosa T1a Tumour invades lamina propria or muscularis mucosase T1b Tumour invades submucosa
T2	Tumour invades muscularis propria or > 1cm	Tumour invades muscularis propria
T3	Tumour invades pancreas or retroperitoneum (for duodenum, ampulla and proximal jejunum) Tumour invades serosa (for lower jejunum and ileum)	Tumour invades subserosa, or non-peritonealized perimuscular tissue (mesentery or retroperitoneum) with extension of 2cm or less
T4	Tumour invades peritoneum or other organs	Tumour perforates visceral peritoneum or directly invades other organs or structures (includes other loops of small intestine, mesentery, or retroperitoneum more than 2cm and abdominal wall by way of serosa; for duodenum only, invasion of pancreas)
N – regional lymph nodes		
NX	Regional lymph node status cannot be assessed	
N0	No regional lymph node metastases	
N1	Regional lymph node metastases	
M – distant metastases		
MX	Distant metastases cannot be assessed	
M0	No distant metastases	
M1	Distant metastases	

Table 18 - Proposal for a pTNM classification for neuroendocrine tumours of the duodenum/ampulla/jejunum and ileum; adapted from [71, 72]

Stage	T	N	M
Stage 1	T1	N0	M0
Stage 2a	T2	N0	M0
Stage 2b	T3	N0	M0
Stage 3a	T4	N0	M0
Stage 3b	Any T	N1	M0
Stage 4	Any T	Any N	M1

Table 19 - Proposal for disease staging for neuroendocrine tumours of the duodenum/ampulla/jejunum and ileum; adapted from [77]

4.3.6 Neuroendocrine tumours of the appendix

Classifying appendiceal neuroendocrine tumours is slightly different than classifying other NETs in the digestive tract (see **Table 20**). In particular, instead of poorly-differentiated carcinomas, mixed exocrine-neuroendocrine carcinomas (goblet cell carinoid/carcinoma) belong to the WHO-group 3. [62]

These tumours are the first or second frequent NETs in the gastrointestinal tract. Remarkably, the age peak for NETs of the appendix belonging to WHO-group 1 and 2 (up to 95%) is far earlier than those of other NETs, at 15 to 25 years. Goblet-cell carcinomas are found later in life with a peak in the 5th and 7th decade of life. There is very likely a female preponderance. [90]

Carcinoid-syndrome is only found in rare cases. [77]

Pathological findings

Well-differentiated tumours/carcinomas

70% of appendiceal NETs are found at the tip of the appendix, nearly always solitary. The tumours are composed of EC-cells expressing serotonin and have a low mitotic rate. Risk of lymph-node metastases is definitely associated with size (1-2cm: 1%, >2cm 30%). Localisation at the base of the appendix might have higher risk of tumour recurrence compared to localisation at the tip. has Prognostic value of invasion of the mesoappendix is still in discussion: Invasion of the subserosa and mesoappendix <3mm might not worsen the prognosis whereas invasion of the mesoappendix >3mm (deep invasion) and angioinvasion have definite bad prognostic markers. 5-year survival time is 83% for all stages, 94% for regional disease and only 31% for distant metastases. [90]

Mixed exocrine-neuroendocrine carcinomas

Synonyms for this tumour are goblet cell carcinoids (GCC), adenocarcinoids or mucinous adenocarcinoids. As mentioned above, the origin of all subtypes of epithelial cells is a single multipotent cell. This tumour consists of cells with different types of differentiation – both goblet cells and endocrine cells. Thus, both cells positive for chromogranin A/synaptophysin and cells showing ring-like structures, positive for mucicarmine can be found. Prognosis is worse than those for well-differentiated NETs, with an overall 5-year survival of 76%. Whereas the prognostic value of size is equally to well-differentiated NETs, both serosa- and mesoappendix invasion appear to be bad prognostic markers. [90]

Clinical findings

Appendiceal NETs are most often found because of symptoms of acute appendicitis, especially pain in the right lower quadrant of the abdomen. They are also detected intraoperatively during pelvic surgery or cholecystectomy by chance. Carcinoid-syndrome is extremely rare. [90]

1	**Well-differentiated neuroendocrine tumour (carcinoid)** Benign: non-functioning, confined to appendiceal wall, non-angioinvasive, ≤ 2cm • Serotonin-producing tumour • Enteroglucagon-producing tumour Benign or low grade malignant (uncertain malignant potential): non-functioning, invading the mesoappendix, angioinvasive, >2cm
2	**Well-differentiated neuroendocrine carcinoma (malignant carcinoid)** Low grade malignant: infiltrating deeply into the mesoappendix, >2,5cm or with metastases • Non-functioning or functioning serotonin-producing carcinoma (with carcinoid syndrome)
3	**Mixed exocrine-neuroendocrine carcinoma** Low grade malignant: Goblet cell carcinoma

Table 20 - Overview of the classification of neuroendocrine tumours of the appendix; taken from [62]

Abbreviation	Characteristics	
T - primary tumour; For any T add (m) for multiple tumours	ENETS	AJCC/UICC
TX	Primary tumour cannot be assessed	Primary tumour cannot be assessed
T0	No evidence of primary tumour	No evidence of primary tumour
T1	Tumour ≤1cm, invading submucosa and muscularis propria	Tumour ≤ 2cm in greatest dimension T1a Tumour ≤ 1cm in greatest dimension T1b Tumour 1-2cm
T2	Tumour ≤2cm invading submucuosa, muscularis propria and/or minimally (up to 3mm) subserosa/mesoappendix	Tumour more than 2cm but not more than 4cm or with extension to the coecum
T3	Tumour >2cm and/or extensive (more than 3mm) invasion of subserosa/mesoappendix	Tumour more than 4cm or with extension to the ileum
T4	Tumour invades peritoneum/other organs	Tumour perforates peritoneum or invades other adjacent organs or structures, e.g. abdominal wall or skeletal muscle
N – regional lymph nodes		
NX	Regional lymph node status cannot be assessed	
N0	No regional lymph node metastases	
N1	Regional lymph node metastases	
M – distant metastases		
MX	Distant metastases cannot be assessed	
M0	No distant metastases	
M1	Distant metastases	

Table 21 - Proposal for a pTNM classification for neuroendocrine tumours of the appendix; taken from [71, 72]

Stage	T	N	M
Stage 1	T1	N0	M0
Stage 2a	T2	N0	M0
Stage 2b	T3	N0	M0
Stage 3a	T4	N0	M0
Stage 3b	Any T	N1	M0
Stage 4	Any T	Any N	M1

Table 22 - Proposal for disease staging by ENETS of neuroendocrine tumours of the appendix; taken from [77]

Stage	T	N	M
Stage 1	T1	N0	M0
Stage 2	T2, T3	N0	M0
Stage 3	T4	N0	M0
	Any T	N1	M0
Stage 4	Any T	Any N	M1

Table 23 – Proposal for disease staging by AJCC/UICC of neuroendocrine tumours of the appendix, taken from [72]

4.3.7 Neuroendocrine tumours of the colon and rectum

NETs of the colon and rectum are responsible for 8% and 27% of all digestive neuroendocrine tumours. Both tumours differ in their biological behaviour because: colon tumours have already metastasized often at diagnosis, rectal tumours are mostly small, without metastases. Therefore prognosis of NETs in the colon is bad with 5-year survival rate of 40-70%, whereas rectal NETs show a 5-year survival rate of 75-88%. Functioning NETs are very rare for both sites, just like poorly-differentiated carcinomas.[91]

An association to chronic inflammatory bowel diseases is discussed.[91] Furthermore many patients develop a colorectal adenocarcinoma at the same time or some years after diagnosis, especially for poorly-differentiated NETs. Similar risk factors for adenocarcinomas and NETs have therefore been discussed.[77]

Pathological findings

Well-differentiated tumours/carcinomas

Colon NETs can be found in the coecal region most often. *Recently, "microcarcinoids" (0.5 to 1.5mm in size) have been described in polypous colonic adenomas* [77]. Rectal NETs often are polypoid submucosal lesions, mostly smaller than 1cm. [77]

The immunohistochemical profiles of the tumour cells are different at each site. Whereas coecal NETs stain for synaptophysin, chromogranin A and serotonin, rectal carcinoids express synaptophysin but not chromogranin A and additional glucagon, glicentin and/or pancreatic polypeptide. [77]

Risk factors for metastases are both size >2cm and invasion of the muscularis propria. If rectal NETs are smaller than 1cm, metastases are very unlikely. A size of 1-2cm is associated with a risk for metastases of approximately 5%. [77]

Poorly-differentiated carcinomas

The cells are either very small or large but usually have high mitotic indices and necrosis. chromogranin A is only rarely expressed. The tumours are large at the time of diagnosis (average 4.9cm). Sufficient information about survival rates is lacking (low frequency). [77]

Clinical findings

Symptoms for colonic carcinoids are similar to adenocarcinomas: Diarrhea, abdominal pain, blood loss (resulting in anemia) and weight loss. Severe gastrointestinal bleeding and bowel obstruction can occur as well. [91]

Rectal carcinoids are usually incidental findings during endoscopy of the rectum. Blood per rectum and pain may be possible symptoms. [91]

Carcinoid-syndrome of functioning NETs is hardly ever found. [91]

Abbreviation	Characteristics	
T - primary tumour; For any T add (m) for multiple tumours	ENETS	AJCC/UICC
TX	Primary tumour cannot be assessed	Primary tumour cannot be assessed
T0	No evidence of primary tumour	No evidence of primary tumour
T1	Tumour invades mucosa or submucosa T1a size <1cm T1b size 1-2cm	Tumour invades lamina propria or submucosa and is ≤ 2cm in size T1a Tumour < 1cm in greatest dimension T1b Tumour 1-2cm
T2	Tumour invades muscularis propria or size >2cm	Tumour invades muscularis propria or size >2cm
T3	Tumour invades subserosa/pericolic/perirectal fatty tissue	Tumour invades subserosa, or non-peritonealized pericolic or perirectal tissues
T4	Tumour directly invades other organs/structures and/or perforates visceral peritoneum	Tumour perforates peritoneum or invades other organs
N – regional lymph nodes		
NX	Regional lymph node status cannot be assessed	
N0	No regional lymph node metastases	
N1	Regional lymph node metastases	
M – distant metastases		
MX	Distant metastases cannot be assessed	
M0	No distant metastases	
M1	Distant metastases	

Table 24 - Proposal for a pTNM classification of neuroendocrine tumours of the colon and rectum; taken from [71, 72]

Stage	T	N	M
Stage 1a	T1a	N0	M0
Stage 1b	T1b	N0	M0
Stage 2a	T2	N0	M0
Stage 2b	T3	N0	M0
Stage 3a	T4	N0	M0
Stage 3b	Any T	N1	M0
Stage 4	Any T	Any N	M1

Table 25 - Proposal for disease staging of neuroendocrine tumours of the colon and rectum; taken from [77]

4.4 Hereditary tumour syndromes associated with neuroendocrine tumours of the gastrointestinal tract

4.4.1 Multiple endocrine neoplasia type 1 (MEN1)

Multiple endocrine neoplasia type 1 (synonym Wermer's disease) is an autosomal dominant inherited disease due to a mutation of MEN1-gene with a prevelance of about 1/30000. Approx. 10% of patients have spontaneous mutations without family history. MEN1 mainly effects endocrine tissues including the parathyroid (95% parathyroid adenoma), the gastro-enteropancreatic neuroendocrine cells (up to 60%, see below), the adrenals (non-functioning tumours of the cortex in up to 30%, rare cases of cancer; pheochromocytoma 1%), the anterior pituitary (prolactinoma 25%, others 10-20%) and sometimes but rarely, the lung (bronchial NETs 4%) and the thymus (NET in up to 2%). In addition, it is associated with tumours of the connective tissue including facial angiofibroma (85%), collagenoma (70%), lipoma (30%), leiomyoma and meningeoma (up to 5%). [92]

The localizations of manifestation in the digestive tract include the stomach, the duodenum and the pancreas. 20-60% of patients show ZES-syndrome due to multiple duodenal gastrinomas. They are usually small (0,3 to 5mm); nonetheless these tumours tend to metastasize into regional lymph nodes early. Additionally, multiple locations of somatostatin-cell hyperplasia and tumours can be found in the duodenum. In the stomach there might be multiple gastric NETs (Type 2) often associated with ECL-hyperplasia. Metastases of these tumours are seldom. [92]

In 30-75% of cases, the pancreas harbours numerous microadenomas (up to 5mm) and often additionally one ore more macroadenomas (>5mm). The tumour cells are multihormonal (most often expressing glucagon and PP). 10-25% of patients develop an insulinoma, with risk of metastases lower than 10%. [92]

4.4.2 Neurofibromatosis type 1 (NF1)

Neurofibromatosis Typ 1 is an autosomal-dominant inherited syndrome too. It is caused by a defect in NF1 – gene. The major manifestations of NF1 neurofibromas are café au lait patches of the skin, endocrine tumours, bone dysplasia, optic nerve and brain stem gliomas and malignant nerve sheath tumours. Endocrine tumours include pheochromocytomas, hyperparathyroidism, medullary thyroid cancer and NETs of duodenum (in only 1%). They are localised in the periampullary region and often stain for somatostatin (no case of somatostatinoma syndrome ever reported). These tumours show metastases in approx. 20%. [92]

4.4.3 Von Hippel-Lindau disease (VHL)

Von Hippel-Lindau disease is an autosomal-dominant disease too. This syndrome includes renal clear cell carcinoma, hemangioblastoma, pheochromocytoma, lesions of the pancreas (50-77%; mostly cystic) and NETs of the pancreas (5-17%). These tumours rarely express hormones; almost all are non-functioning, 10-20% of patients present with metastases. [92]

4.4.4 Tuberous sclerosis complex

The tuberous sclerosis complex includes hamartomatous lesions in brain, skin, eyes, heart, lungs, kidneys resulting in epilepsy, mental retardation or autism. It is a autosomal-dominant disease, with a prevalence of 1:10000. In only 1% it is associated with NETs of the pancreas, either insulinomas or functionally inactive tumours. [92]

4.5 Diagnostic tools

Depending on the localisation, there are multiple options for detecting and diagnosing neuroendocrine tumours of the gastrointestinal tract. These include both conventional diagnostic tools such as CT-scan or MRI or upper gastrointestinal endoscopy/colonoscopy, and also highly specialised methods such as somatostatin-receptor-scintigraphy or biochemical serum investigations such as chromogranin A, hormones and specialised functional tests to confirm the diagnosis of a functional neuroendocrine tumour (secretin-test, 72h-hour-fast etc.). Each imaging technique has to be validated of course by histological evaluation of tumour cells as describe above.

4.5.1 Imaging techniques

Endoscopy

Upper gastrointestinal endoscopy and colonoscopy may be of increasing importance in diagnosing neuroendocrine tumours. Gastric and duodenal NETs especially can often be assessed and evaluated by gastroscopy due to the fact that radiological methods (CT, MRI) are insufficient for displaying small lesions in the upper gastrointestinal tract. With rising numbers of gastroscopies and coloscopies performed routinely, this may lead to higher incidence rates for gastric NETs as suspected by Klöppel [77] and in the recent ENETs guidelines [78]. Recto-colonoscopy is of similar importance for NETs of the colon and rectum. Both gastroscopy and colonoscopy can also be used to obtain biopsies of tumours.

Ultrasound

Abdominal ultrasound (± contrast agent) is used mainly for imaging of the liver (especially in searching for metastases), the pancreas and great abdominal masses. Doppler and Duplex-sonography help to look for a tumour's blood support. Ultrasound is also used intraoperatively. [78-84, 86, 88-90]
Additionally, endoscopical ultrasound (EUS) is essential, especially for imaging of the gastric and duodenal wall (measuring the tumour-infiltration depth) but also the pancreas' head for very small lesions (probably the most sensitive imaging technique for insulinoma). Lastly, rectal (endoanal) ultrasound is a very accurate tool for evaluating rectal NETs. [78-84, 86, 88-90]

Computed Tomography (CT) and Magnetic Resonance Imaging (MRI)

CT-Scan (performed as multi-slice triple phase CT; including CT colonography) and MRI (including MR-cholangiopancreatography and –angiography) are invaluable for tumour-staging. Whereas CT has probably advantages for imaging thorax and abdomen, MRI may be superior for the liver, pancreas and the pelvis. [78-84, 86, 88-90]

Somatostatin-receptor Scintigraphy - ^{111}In-DTPA Octreotide Scanning (Octreo-Scan)

Octreotid-Scan is a method used to visualise tumours expressing somatostatin-receptors (SSTR). As mentioned, above there are 5 subtypes of SSTR. Subtype 2 and 5 are expressed most often in gastrointestinal neuroendocrine tumours and octreotide (a synthetic 8-amino-acid somatostatin-analogue) binds especially to these receptors. For tumours expressing somatostatin-receptors, this is a very sensitive tool and visualizes even small lesions. [78-84, 86, 88-90]

Positron-Emission-Tomography (PET) and PET-CT

Especially PET-CT is a very new and promising tool for localising even the smallest neuroendocrine tumours. Various tracers have been used: C-5-HTP and 18F-Dopa are very important for highly-differentiated tumours (with uptake of amines) whereas 18F-fluorodeoxyglucose (18-F-FDG) is used for poorly-differentiated tumours. 68Ga-DOTA-DPhe1-Tyr3-octreotide (68Ga-DOTATOC) is a tracer binding to somatostatin-receptors and therefore can be used alternatively for both Octreotide-Scan and PET. According to recent analyses, this method may be the optimum approach for visualising NETs. [78-84, 86, 88-90]

4.5.2 Laboratory tests

Serum concentration of Chromogranin A can be used as general marker for neuroendocrine tumours. It is not specific for the gastrointestinal tract only since it is also elevated in neuroendocrine tumours of e.g. the lung or any other tissue. The level is correlated with extension and prognosis of a neuroendocrine tumour [61, 93]. However, use of chromogranin A depends on the quality of the used assay, in particular, the antibodies, which still have not been standardised. [93]

Further laboratory tests are specific for each tumour site and suspected hormonal syndrome:

Fasting serum gastrin levels, measured after withdrawal of proton pump inhibitors for at least 1 week, are elevated in both gastric NETs and gastrinomas. But in order to distinguish between these tumours, gastric pH has to be measured as well (type 1 gastric NETs high pH, type 2 and gastrinoma low pH). If Gastrin levels are greater than 1000pg/ml, no further testing is needed if a gastrinoma is suspected. Levels below have to be confirmed by the secretin-test. Secretin is injected 1U/kg and gastrin is measured several times in a short interval. A twofold increase in serum gastrin indicates a ZES caused by a gastrinoma. [78, 80, 86, 93]

Insulin, Pro-Insulin and C-peptide are relevant parameters for insulinomas. These parameters are assessed several times during a 72h-fasting. Insulin, its precursors and metabolites are elevated, whereas blood glucose that falls below 40 mg/dl causes neurological symptoms (Index insulin:blood-glucose >0.3; Normally <0.25). [83, 86, 93]

For patients suffering for small-intestine NETs, Serotonin serum levels and additional further peptides secreted by EC-cells (Bradykinin, Neurokinin, Substance P etc.) can be measured. 24h-urine-excretion of 5-hydroxy-indolic-acetic acid (5-HIAA) is elevated in patients with serotonin-producing tumours, including those suffering from carcinoid-syndrome. Some authors recommend stimulation-test with pentagastrin (0.06 mg/kg) causing a rise in serum serotonin levels. [86, 88, 93]

Further hormones should be assessed in serum, depending on clinical symptoms (e.g. Glucagon, VIP, somatostatin, PP).

4.6 Therapeutic options

As with nearly any other neoplastic disease, the only curative therapy is complete tumour resection. However, this is often simply not possible especially due to late diagnosis with absence of symptoms – the tumour itself has either metastasised or its local infiltration is too extensive. Compared to other carcinomas, in neuroendocrine tumours, there are several therapeutic options to control progressive stages of disease including peptide radio-receptor therapy or therapy with somatostatin analogues for example.

The most important treatment options of neuroendocrine tumours are summarized briefly in the following section.

4.6.1 Interventional techniques

Endoscopy

NETs are now diagnosed more often due to the increasing frequency of endoscopies of the upper and lower intestinal tract especially gastric, duodenal, colonic and rectal ones. Endoscopy implements the possibility not only to take biopsies of suspect tissues but also to remove small lesions such as polypoid tumours completely. This is an important option especially for early tumour stages. In addition, endoscopical mucosectomy can be performed even for multiple NETs (up to 6) not infiltrating underlying structures, especially gastric NETs Type 1 and 2. [78]

Surgery

Surgery is the therapy of choice, whenever complete tumour resection is possible and metastases are absent. Only complete tumour resection (R0) is potentially curative. The presence of hepatic metastases (distant metastases) needs careful evaluation - whether metastases can be operated on, depending on differentiation of the tumour (only well-differentiated!), distribution of metastases, patient's general condition and the absence of both extra-abdominal metastases and of peritoneal carcinomatosis. If these conditions are fulfilled, surgery improves survival significantly. Even liver transplantation may be an option for a few selected patients to cure the disease. However this procedure has only been performed about 150 times worldwide and is still controversial since long-term data are lacking. [86, 94, 95]

Resection of metastases leaving the primary tumour is not recommended. [94]

For appendical tumours, there are special recommendations. Tumours smaller than 2cm can most often be cured with appendectomy alone; patients with a tumour size of more than 2cm and deep mesoappendiceal invasion should be treated with a right hemicolectomy. [86, 94, 95]

Palliative surgery (tumour debulking) is needed whenever a tumour causes bowel obstruction or kinking – sometimes the first symptom of a neuroendocrine tumour of the small intestine. [86, 94, 95]

Peptide-receptor-radio-therapy (PRRT)

Peptide-receptor-radio-therapy (also called Peptide-radioreceptor-therapy) is an interesting new therapy concept for NETs. The most important precondition for using this method is that the tumour expresses peptide-receptors. The principle of this radiotherapy is intuitive: A radioactive substance (radionuclide; e.g. yttrium, lutetium) is bound via a complexing agent (DOTA, DTPA) to a ligand binding to a peptide receptor (an "analogue" to its real ligand; e.g. octreotide). The radiation emitted from the radionuclide destroys cells binding the ligand. Although every peptide-receptor expressed on a tumour cell can hypothetically be used, only octreotide and lanreotide (both somatostatin analogues, binding mainly to sst-2 and -5 receptors) are available at the moment. The various procedures are DOTATOC (90Y-DOTA-Octreotide), DOTA-TATE (177Lu-DOTA-Octreotate), DTPA-OC (111In-DTPA-Octreotide) or DOTA-Lanreotide (90Y-DOTA-Lanreotide). [86, 94, 95]

PRRT is only performed in palliative settings in patients with multiple (liver) metastases when surgery is not possible. Data provide evidence that this therapy can at least stabilise the disease. However complete remission is rare. [86, 94, 95]

Ablative techniques for liver metastases

Currently there are a handful of different ablative techniques available for liver metastases of neuroendocrine carcinomas. Data is limited because of the little number of cases fulfilling criteria for ablative techniques (surgery not indicated because of multiple metastases or patient's general condition) – therefore experience comes mainly from ablation of other tumours (adenocarcinomas). Radiofrequency ablation uses electricity (either percutaneous or during laparoscopy) to destroy tumour cells, Laser-induced thermotherapy. Cryotherapy uses temperature to reduce tumour-mass, selective ethanol injection (percutaneous) is a chemical way and brachytherapy uses radioactive energy for diminishing metastases. [86, 94, 95]

Ablative techniques can also be used intraoperatively when e.g. the primary tumour has to be resected but liver metastases cannot be operated on. [86, 94, 95]

Chemoembolisation

Chemoembolisation is also performed only in progressive tumour disease if surgical resection of the liver metastases is not possible. There are two procedures for chemoembolisation of liver metastases in NETs: Trans-catheter arterial embolisation (TAE) or trans-catheter arterial chemoembolisation (TACE). In both techniques hepatic arteriography is used to search for vessels supplying the metastases. If these can be detected, they are either occluded with embolic particles only (TAE) or embolisation is performed after injection of a cytostatic agent such as doxorubicin or streptozotocin (TACE). [86, 94, 95]

4.6.2 Medical therapies

Conservative therapies for neuroendocrine tumours include somatostatin-analogue-therapy, interferon-therapy and chemotherapy. The first two are sometimes called biotherapy – their primary aim is to control/reduce both tumour symptoms due to hormonal hypersecretion and tumour growth.
Both biotherapies can be combined but clinical trials show that there is hardly any difference to monotherapy. Combination-therapy should be avoided because there is no advantage compared to monotherapy and due to the high costs. [86, 94, 95]
Biotherapy is indicated mainly in well-differentiated carcinoma with hormonal activity to control symptoms and stabilise disease. [86, 94, 95]

Somatostatin analogues (SSA)

As mentioned in chapter 2.3.2, somatostatin inhibits both hormonal secretion and cell growth. Its actions are mediated via somatostatin-receptors – currently 5 subtypes are known (sst1 – 5). Neuroenendocrine tumours often show a higher expression of somatostatin-receptors than normal neuroendocrine cells, although often not homogenously. Therefore somatostatin-analogues are used to activate somatostatin-receptors expressed on the surface of neuroendocrine tumour cells. [86, 94, 95]
There a two approved analogues: Octreotide and lanreotide. Both of them bind mainly to sst-2 and -5. Their half-life time is longer than that of somatostatin itself – however e.g. octreotide has to be injected 3-times a day. Therefore there are depot-forms for intramuscular injection (lanreotide long-lasting and octreotide long-acting repeatable [LAR]) that have to be administered every two to six weeks only. Another analogue, pasireotide, is currently under clinical investigation. Pasireotide binds to sst 1-3 and -5 and might therefore be superior to the other analogues. [86, 94, 95]
SSA-therapy is used in patients with hormonally active tumours. It is effective for controlling symptoms in carcinoid-syndrome, insulinoma, VIPoma and Glucagonoma. Somatostatin-analogues may also stabilise tumour growth. [86, 94, 95]

Use of somatostatin-analogues is mainly limited by development of tachyphylaxis. The time it takes to be ineffective can be as long as a few weeks to many years. Side-effects are abdominal discomfort, steatorrhea due to inhibition of exocrine pancreas-secretion, cholestasis and cholecystolithiasis. Vitamin-B12 levels may decline too (inhibition of intrinsic factor secretion). [86, 94, 95]

Interferon

Interferon-α 2a or 2b (IFN) has been used for treating solid tumours. It has multiple effects that include tumour suppression, inhibition of cell-cycle, induction of apoptosis, inhibition of protein-synthesis and enhanced expression of MHC1-antigens on the surface of tumour cells. The latter effect results in a higher activity of cytotoxic T-cells against tumour cells, destroying them. [86, 94, 95]

Similar to SSA-therapy, Interferon is able to stabilise tumour growth, although it can hardly bring complete tumour remission. It is also able to control symptoms due to hormonal overexpression – but especially for carcinoid syndrome, its effects are less convincing than with SSA. [86, 94, 95]

Interferon is administered subcutaneously, either 3 times a week or once weekly using pegylated interferon. Side effects include flu-like symptoms (nearly always), loss of appetite and weight, fatigue, hepatotoxicity and bone marrow suppression (anemia, leuko- and thrombocytopenia). [86, 94, 95]

Chemotherapy

Systemic chemotherapy is used mainly for metastatic neuroendocrine tumours of the stomach, duodenum and pancreas while results for other sites (small intestine, large intestine) are unsatisfying. Indications to start chemotherapy are low-differentiated tumours with metastases but also therapy failure during other treatments (biotherapy). [86, 94, 95]

Therapy concepts are always combination-therapies since monotherapies appear to be less effective. Streptozocin is most often combined with 5-Fluoruracil (5-FU), cyclophosphamid, dacarbazin or doxorubicin, sometimes even as triplet-therapy. Low-differentiated carcinomas are treated with etoposid and cisplatin. [86, 94, 95]

Currently, new substances are under intensive investigation. Both tyrosine-kinase inhibitors (e.g. imatinib, sunitimib) and antiangiogeneic agents (e.g. endostatin, bevacuzimab, thalidomide) may provide new therapy options, maybe in combination with biotherapy. [86, 94, 95]

4.7 Incidence in other countries

Numerous incidence studies were published in the past years. To the author's knowledge, nearly all of them are based on data coming exclusively from cancer registers and therefore are retrospective studies. Only one study by Berge et al[96] from Sweden, an autopsy study, is not based on database entries but on clinical investigation.

In the following section, 4 incidence studies - 2 from the USA, 1 from Sweden and 1 from Switzerland are presented briefly as examples either because they are often cited in literature or they present special information:

- A paper by J.D. Godwin[97] from the USA published in 1974 is of special interest. It was one of the incidence studies published first and for many years, it was considered the "standard" paper concerning the incidence of NETs in the gastrointestinal tract.
- Modlin et al[98] published another database analysis in 2003, which is most recognized and found in literature so far - mainly because of the high number of tumours recorded.
- The Swedish study by Hemminki et al[99] from 2001 presents incidence data for a country very similar to Austria in size and composition of population and similar also in accessibility and quality of health care system.
- Swiss data from 2000 by Levi et al[100] will be mentioned because this study is the only one that distinguishes between benign and malignant neuroendocrine tumours.

4.7.1 Godwin II JD - Carcinoid Tumours – An Analysis of 2837 Cases

This study from 1974 was based on two different databases run by the National Cancer Institute (NCI) of the USA. Combined, the End Result Group (ERG) database and the Third National Cancer Survey (TNCS) database collected data about multiple kinds of cancer. Patients had been treated in about 100 different hospitals all around the USA (10% of US-population). [97]

Godwin analysed neuroendocrine tumours (the author calls them carcinoids) fulfilling the inclusion criteria: date of diagnosis between 1950 and 1969 and confirmation of diagnosis by histology (no further information about the criteria). The study did not include data about gastrointestinal NETs only but also bronchopulmonary NETs (10-14% of all NETs; the latter being left out in this summary).

Godwin himself states in the paper that benign NETs are probably reported too seldom for two reasons: First - regarding the ERG database: patients with benign NETs had to agree to being included into the database (whereas they were included automatically for malignant ones) Second, in TNCS, no benign lesions were collected at all. However Godwin argues that only 2% of NETs were classified as benign during the study period and therefore that fact would not bias the results. [97]

The results were given separately for male, female, blacks and whites. Godwin reports a tendency towards black and male patients with the important exception of appendiceal NETs (female preponderance). Because the US-white population is best comparable to the Austrian population, the following data includes only white US-citizens (summed up in **Table 26**). Summarizing the age-adjusted incidence rates of gastrointestinal NETs for white males were 1.00/100000/year and for white females 1.32/100000/year. In men, the most frequent localisation of a GI-NETs turned out in the small intestine followed by the appendix, whereas for women it is the opposite. No case was reported in the pancreas or Meckel Diverticulum. [97]

Site	White males	White females
Stomach	0.03	0.02
Small intestine	0.48	0.28
Colon except appendix	0.11	0.07
Appendix	0.25	0.79
Rectum and rectosigmoid	0.14	0.15
Total	**1.01**	**1.33**

Table 26 - Age-adjusted incidence rates* n/100000/year for the white US-population for the years 1950-69[97]
* No information about how age-adjusted incidence rates were calculated

4.7.2 Modlin IM - A 5-Decade Analysis of 13715 Carcinoid Tumors

This study from 2003 was based on data combinig both Godwin's work (see above) and another registry. Godwin's work (see above) and another registry - the Surveillance, Epidemiology and End result (SEER) database (again run by the NCI) for the years 1973-1999. 13715 neuroendocrine tumours (again the author calls them "carcinoid tumours") could be analysed in total; 2837 from Godwin's analysis and another 10878 from the SEER database. About 14% of the US-population was covered using these databases, the sample again being representative for the whole US-population.
The study covers the years 1950 to 1999. Similar to Godwin's work, no information is given about how the diagnosis "neuroendocrine tumour" was confirmed or how the tumours were classified. Besides, Modlin remarks that up to 1986, only malignant NETs were reported. Like Godwin, he argues that most of NETs were malignant anyway. The study includes also all bronchopulmonary NETs diagnosed. [98]
Data are split up not only by gender and the different races present in the US-population (whites, blacks, hispancis, asians) but also by the different databases combined in the study (TNCS, early SEER [1973-1991], late SEER [1992-1999]). In the following only gastrointestinal NETs from the late SEER will be mentioned. [98]
Modlin found a slightly higher affliction of blacks (black:white ratio 1.32) and of asians (asian:non-asian ratio 1.84). Conversely, NETs were reported less in hispanics (hispanic:non-hispanic ratio 0.31). The male:female ratio was 1.03. [98]

The overall age-adjusted incidence rate for whites from 1992-1999 were 1.80/100000/year for males and 1.52/100000/year for females. [98]

In comparing the sites of the tumours the small intestine was found most often, followed by rectum and colon, regardless of gender. **Table 27** summarises the data for white population in the U.S. from 1992-1999. [98]

Site	White male	White females
Stomach	0.12	0.18
Small intestine	0.88	0.63
Appendix	0.06	0.08
Colon	0.21	0.18
Rectum and rectosigmoid junction	0.41	0.35
Liver	0.02	0.01
Gallbladder	0.01	0.01
Other biliary	0.01	0.01
Pancreas	0.02	0.01
Digestive tract, NOS	0.06	0.06
Total	1.80	1.52

Table 27 – Age adjusted incidence rates* n/100000/year for the white US-population for the years 1992-1999
* Using 1992-2000 US standard population

4.7.3 Hemminiki K - Incidence Trends and Risk Factors of Carcinoid Tumors

This study from 2001 was based upon the Swedish Family-Cancer Database (from 1958 to 1998) and includes 5184 neuroendocrine tumours (author: carcinoid tumours). The Swedish Family Cancer Database records all cases of cancer in Sweden (close to 100% of population; totalling approximately 10 million people). This study includes bronchopulmonary NETs too (again excluded in the following). Hemminki neither mentions benign NETs nor gives information about the confirmation of diagnoses and the classification of the tumours. [99]

Incidence rates were calculated for the years 1983-1999. Females patients had NETs in the appendix most often, whereas in male patients, gastrointestinal NETs were most often found in the small intestine,. The median age was lowest for appendiceal tumours (32 years male, 31 years female). Detailed data about pancreas and liver tumours are missing. These could be included in a subgroup called "others". However, because this group may also include urogenital and other NETs, they are excluded in this summary. The standardized incidence rate for NETs in the gastrointestinal tract for men was 1.6/10000/year and for women 1.9/10000/year. Further details are given in **Table 28**. [99]

Site	Men*	Median age (m)	Women*	Median age (f)
Stomach	0.1	60	0.1	63
Small intestine	0.8	66	0.6	66
Appendix	0.4	32	0.8	31
Colon	0.1	61	0.2	48
Rectum	0.2	57	0.2	52
Total	**1.6**		**1.9**	

Table 28 – Age-adjusted* incidence rates n/100000/year for the Swedish population for the years 1983-1998.
* No information about which standard population was used

4.7.4 Levi F - Epidemiology of carcinoid neoplasms in Vaud, Switzerland, 1974-97

This study from 2000 was absed on date from Canton Vaud is a region of Switzerland, having approximately 57000 inhabitants. Data were collected using the Vaud Cancer Registry data file, which includes both all malignant neoplasms but also selected non-malignant or precancerous lesions (incl. benign NETs). However, no information is given about the confirmation of diagnosis and the classification scheme of NETs. [100]

Data are split into years 1974-1985 and 1986-1997. In this summary, only data for the period 1986 to 1997 are used, again excluding bronchopulmonary NETs. Appendiceal tumours are included into colorectal NETs. No data are given for pancreas and liver NETs (summed up in "others"?).

141 of 174 (81%) colorectal tumours and 14 of 19 (74%) were benign, showing a preponderance for benign tumours for these sites. However, only 44 of 116 (38%) small intestinal NETs were classified as benign. Colorectal NETs were found most often, followed by small intestine NETs and stomach NETs. [100]

The age-adjusted standardised incidence rate for gastrointestinal NETs was 2,05 for male and 2,17 for female patients [100]. Detailed data are given in **Table 29**.

Site	Male	Female
Stomach	0.17	0.03
Small intestine	0.90	0.44
Colon/rectum	0.98	1.70
Total	**2.05**	**2.17**

Table 29 – Age-adjusted standardised incidence rates* n/100000/year for Canton Vaud, Switzerland for the years 1974-1997
* Using world standard population (Doll and Smith 1987)

5. Original Research

5.1 Aims of the study

- To determine the incidence of gastroenteropancreatic neuroendocrine tumours in Austria

- To determine the incidence of gastroenteropancreatic neuroendocrine tumours in a central European country with a highly developed medical training and social framework based on a strict immunohistochemical protocol which applies the current WHO-Classification[63]

- To apply the recent ENETs guidelines for staging and grading [70, 71] to an incidence survey

- To identify the methods of diagnosis of GEP-NETs in everyday routine in Austria

- To describe the clinical presentation at initial diagnosis of GEP-NETs (incl. symptoms, presence of metastasis)

- To collect information about practice of treatment of GEP-NETs in Austria

5.2 Materials and Methods

The trial was designed as a prospective survey and divided into two phases (parts). The objective of the first phase/part was to collect pathology reports of all tumours diagnosed and classified histologically/immunhistochemically as NETs during one year (01/05/2004 – 30/04/2005) to analyse current data on the Austrian national incidence of GEP NETs.

The objective of the second phase/part was to collect and analyse data on the clinical course concerning symptoms, diagnosis and treatment. (see)

In **Figure 2** the study algorithm is presented. In phase1 pathologists who received neuroendocrine tumours from different hospitals and physicans reported the diagnosis directly to the study center. In phase 2, clinical information was provided to the study center directly from the referring physicians and hospitals.

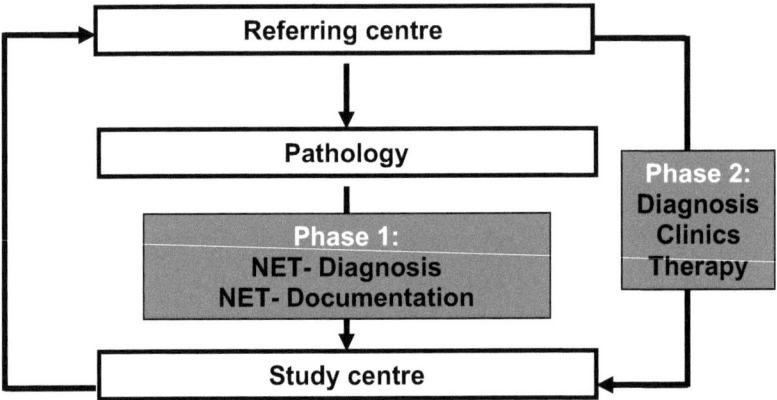

Figure 2 – Study algorithm

5.2.1 Phase 1: Incidence

There are 41 registered departments and institutes of clinical pathology linked to public and private hospitals in Austria (see 8.1). All were invited and 40 participated in this prospective one-year study.

With regard to the study protocol, only patients with NETs located in the gastrointestinal tract and pancreas initially diagnosed within the study period were included in the analysis. Of the 40 participating pathological institutes, 31 reported NETs during the study period and were further evaluated.

The diagnosis of NETs was initially based on typical morphological characteristics [101]. However, the detailed neuroendocrine origin of the tumours was definitively identified using staining for markers of neuroendocrine differentiation, chromogranin A and/or synaptophysin, as recently described [62]. Neuron-specific enolase was not used for characterization as it is not reliable enough [102].

Apart from the histopathological characteristics, additional parameters such as tumour location and the patient's sex and age were documented by the participating institutes and the pathology reports (see 8.3) sent online to the study centre.

Tumour classification

Using the recently published WHO classification [62], the detected NETs were subdivided, irrespective of the site of the primary, into 'well-differentiated' tumours with either 'benign' or 'uncertain' behaviour or as 'well-differentiated' or 'poorly differentiated' neuroendocrine carcinomas.

Neuroendocrine liver tumours were included in the analysis if no other neuroendocrine malignancy outside the abdomen (e.g. lung, ovary) was detected at the time of diagnosis and were therefore assessed as distant metastasis from GEP NETs. For further evaluation of liver tumours, particularly to gain information on location of the primary in the ileum or jejunum, and if adequate amounts of samples were available, tissue was stained immunohistochemically with antibodies against serotonin [103].

The pathological data were supervised by a pathologist, specialised on endocrine pathology (K. Kaserer) and, if questionable, additional immunohistochemical studies were conducted.

5.2.2 Phase 2: Clinical evaluation

In addition to the pathological report, information relating to the patients' attending departments/physicians was documented in order to obtain further details on the clinical course of disease.

A standardized questionnaire was designed comprising approximately 50 clinical and biochemical parameters (see 8.4). The questionnaires were sent to clinicians and attending physicians from 190 departments involved in the care of the patients documented in the pathological reports. The physicians were invited to participate in this part of the study and were asked to complete the questionnaires separately and anonymously for each patient. Contact was made by written invitation and by telephone.

Analysis of clinical data

Patients were integrated into the clinical database only if they had agreed to participate in this part of the study, thus not all patients could be included. As a minimum requirement, information on the mode of diagnosis, presence/absence of metastasis and/or therapeutic information had to be available for integration of a patient's data into the register.

5.2.3 TNM staging and grading based on ENETS definitions

Based on the clinical, surgical and imaging data, the recently published TNM classification and staging system, together with the tumour grading suggested by Rindi et al. [70, 71], were used whenever possible.

5.2.4 Statistical analysis

A Filemaker® database for documentation of patients with NETs was created with records of all pathological and available clinical parameters. SPSS® Version 17.0 was used for statistical analyses. Only patients with tumours defined immunhistochemically as NETs based on rigorous immunohistochemical criteria (definition see above) were selected from the database for the clinical analysis.

Data are described as median and interquartile range (IQR). Age-standardized (=age-adjusted) incidence rates were calculated using Austrian population data published by Statistics Austria. The reference population was based on the world population, as used by the International Agency for Research on Cancer [104] and modified by Doll [105] after Segi [106].

For comparison of the Austrian incidence data to those of the usually cited "Surveillance, Epidemiology, and End Results" (SEER) Program of the National Cancer Institute from the USA [98, 107, 108] the age-adjusted incidence rate was further calculated to the 2000 US standard population [109].

The population-based Austrian cancer registry, which recorded all digestive tract cancers in 2004, was used to compare the incidence of malignant NETs with that of gastrointestinal cancer of various sites of the digestive tract. Austria, located in central Europe, has approximately 8.3 million inhabitants, 10% of whom are foreigners mainly from other countries of the European Union, the former Yugoslavia and Turkey.

P values were calculated using Mann–Whitney U-tests and corrected for multiple testing using the Bonferroni–Holm method. P values < 0.05 were considered significant.

5.2.5 Informed consent

All patients were asked to give informed consent for documentation of their pathological and clinical data. Patients' full names were pseudonymised by the pathologists and attending physicians completing the pathologic report forms or questionaires.

The design of the prospective study, the manner of data collection and the retrospective analysis were approved by the ethics committee of the Medical University of Vienna (Resolution number 157/2005).

5.3 Gastro-entero-pancreatic neuroendocrine tumours - the current incidence and staging based on the WHO and ENETS classification

Original paper 1 – published in

Endocrine-Related Cancer **2010** 17 (4) 909 -918 DOI: 10.1677/ERC-10-0152

Authors: Martin B Niederle (Department of General Surgery, Medical University of Vienna), Monika Hackl (Statistik Austria), Klaus Kaserer (Department of Pathology, Medical University of Vienna) and Bruno Niederle (Department of General Surgery, Medical University of Vienna)

Subtitle: an analysis based on prospectively collected parameters

Short title: Gastrointestinal neuroendocrine tumours

Keywords: Neuroendocrine tumours – digestive tract – incidence – WHO classification – TNM Staging

5.3.1 Abstract

Because incidence data on gastroenteropancreatic neuroendocrine tumors (GEP-NETs) have so far only been retrospectively obtained and based on inhomogeneous material, we conducted a prospective study in Austria collecting all newly diagnosed GEP-NETs during one year. Using the current WHO classification, the TNM staging and Ki67-grading, and the standard diagnostic procedure proposed by the European Neuroendocrine Tumor Society, GEP-NETs from 285 patients (male: 148; female: 137) were recorded. The annual incidence rates were 2.51 per 100,000 inhabitants for men, 2.36 for women. The stomach (23%) was the main site, followed by appendix (21%), small intestine (15%) and rectum (14%). Patients with appendiceal tumours were significantly younger than patients with tumours at any other site. 46.0% were classified as benign, 15.4% as uncertain, 31.9% as well-differentiated malignant and 6.7% as poorly differentiated malignant. Patients with benign or uncertain tumours were significantly younger than patients with malignant tumours. Among the malignant tumours of the digestive tract, 1.49% arose from neuroendocrine cells. For malignant gastrointestinal neuroendocrine tumours the incidence was 0.80 per 100,000: 40.9% were ENETS stage I, 23.8% stage II, 11.6% stage III and 23.8% stage IV. The majority (59.7%) were grade 1, 31.2% grade 2 and 9.1% grade 3.

Neuroendocrine tumours of the digestive tract are more common than previously reported. The majority show benign behaviour, are located in the stomach and are well-differentiated. G3 tumours are very rare.

5.3.2 Introduction

Neuroendocrine tumours (NETs) of the gastrointestinal tract are rare neoplasms and represent a heterogeneous group of tumours with distinct functional and biological behaviour depending on location, tumour size and clinical symptoms [62]. NETs arise from the neuroendocrine cells of the diffuse neuroendocrine system. Located in the oesophagus, stomach, duodenum, pancreas, ileum, jejunum, appendix, colon or rectum, these tumours are summarized as gastroenteropancreatic (GEP) NETs [62]; they were formerly referred to as gastrointestinal carcinoids, a term introduced by Oberndorfer more than 100 years ago [6, 110].

NETs were recently classified according standardized histopathological criteria established by the World Health Organization (WHO)[63]. Irrespective of the site of origin, these endocrine tumours are classified in general as "well-differentiated with benign" or "uncertain", "well-differentiated with low-grade malignant" or "poorly differentiated with high-grade malignant behaviour". The classification is based on particular criteria (size, invasion, Ki-67 index etc.) used to predict a tumour's biological behaviour (benign, malignant) with high probability [62].

Incidence data on GEP NETs are difficult to obtain and are mainly based on national cancer registries. These usually document malignant diseases on the basis of clinical reports, and therefore accurate and relevant analysis of the incidence of GEP NETs may have substantial limitations since the majority of NETs with benign or uncertain clinical course may not be fully incorporated. In addition, such data have usually been collected over an extended period, during which time the definitions of the disease have evolved. Furthermore, information on the incidence of NETs in different sites is not as precisely documented in the national registries as information on adenocarcinoma of the digestive tract.

To our knowledge the rare papers analysing the incidence of NETs are either retrospective database analyses [97, 99, 111] or autopsy studies [112] and lack both the recently recommended standardized histopathological characterization and the current WHO classification of NETs.

The aim of this study was to evaluate the incidence of GEP NETs in a Middle European country (Austria) based on prospectively collected pathological reports, using a standardized histopathological protocol for initial diagnosis. The current WHO recommendations were used for classification [62] and the recently defined criteria of the European Neuroendocrine Tumour Society (ENETS) for staging and grading [70, 71]. In addition, the incidence of malignant GEP NETs was compared with that of other malignant tumours identified in the same parts of the digestive tract.

5.3.3 Methods

The objective of the prospective trial was to collect pathology reports of all tumours diagnosed and classified histologically/immunhistochemically as NETs during one year (01/05/2004 – 30/04/2005) to analyse current data on the Austrian national incidence of GEP NETs.

Incidence

There are 41 registered departments and institutes of clinical pathology linked to public and private hospitals in Austria. All were invited and 40 participated in this prospective one-year study.

With regard to the study protocol, only patients with NETs located in the gastrointestinal tract and pancreas initially diagnosed within the study period were included in the analysis. Of the 40 participating pathological institutes, 31 reported NETs during the study period and were further evaluated.

Tumour definition was initially based on typical morphological characteristics [101]. However, the detailed neuroendocrine origin of the tumours was definitively identified using staining for markers of neuroendocrine differentiation, chromogranin A and/or synaptophysin, as recently described [62]. Neuron-specific enolase was not used for characterization as it is insufficiently reliable [102].

Apart from the histopathological characteristics, additional parameters such as tumour location and the patient's sex and age were documented by the participating institutes and the pathology reports sent online to the study centre.

WHO tumour classification

As published recently [62], the detected NETs were subdivided, irrespective of the site of the primary, into 'well-differentiated' tumours with either 'benign' or 'uncertain' behaviour or as 'well-differentiated' or 'poorly differentiated' neuroendocrine carcinomas.

Neuroendocrine liver tumours were included in the analysis if no other neuroendocrine malignancy outside the abdomen (e.g. lung, ovary) was detected at the time of diagnosis and were therefore assessed as distant metastasis from GEP NETs. For further evaluation of liver tumours, particularly to gain information on location of the primary in the ileum or jejunum, and if adequate amounts of samples were available, tissue was stained immunohistochemically with antibodies against serotonin [103].

The pathological data were supervised by one of the authors (KK) and, if questionable, additional immunohistochemical studies were conducted.

TNM staging and grading based on ENETS definitions

Based on the clinical, surgical and imaging data, the recently published TNM classification and staging system, together with the tumour grading suggested by Rindi et al. [70, 71], were used whenever possible.

Statistical analysis

A Filemaker® database for documentation of patients with NETs was built up, recording all pathological and available clinical parameters. SPSS® Version 17.0 was used for statistical analyses.

Data are described as median and interquartile range (IQR). Age-standardized (=age-adjusted) incidence rates were calculated using Austrian population data published by Statistics Austria. The reference population was based on the world population, as used by the International Agency for Research on Cancer [104] and modified by Doll [105] after [106].

For comparison of the Austrian incidence data to those of the usually cited "Surveillance, Epidemiology, and End Results" (SEER) Program of the National Cancer Institute from the USA [98, 107, 108] the age-adjusted incidence rate was further calculated to the 2000 US standard population [109].

The population-based Austrian cancer registry, which recorded all digestive tract cancers in 2004, was used to compare the incidence of malignant NETs with that of gastrointestinal cancer of various sites of the digestive tract. Austria, in central Europe, has about 8.3 million inhabitants, 10% of whom are foreigners mainly from other countries of the European Union, the former Yugoslavia and Turkey.

P values were calculated using Mann–Whitney U-tests and corrected for multiple testing using the Bonferroni–Holm method. P values < 0.05 were considered significant.

Informed consent

All patients were asked to give informed consent for documentation of their pathological and clinical data. The full names of the patients remained unknown to the study centre.

All patients agreed to participate in the "pathological analysis" but not all agreed to participate in the "clinical" part of the study, thus not all patients could be included. Information on the presence/absence of metastasis had to be available as a minimum requirement for ENETS staging.

The design of the prospective study, the manner of data collection and the retrospective analysis were approved by the ethics committee of the Medical University of Vienna (Resolution number 157/2005).

5.3.4 Results

Incidence

A total of 305 tumours were reported during the 12-month period. Eleven specimens were excluded because the immunohistochemistry was either negative or impossible to assess because of inadequate material; an additional five were excluded because the date of diagnosis was not within the study period; a further three specimens were metastasis in the liver of NETs of other sites (lung: 2, ovary: 1) and one biopsy could not be related to an organ (biopsy of a NET of the abdomen). Thus, 285 NETs located in the gastrointestinal tract were selected from the database and were available for detailed evaluation.

Incidence and biological behaviour of neuroendocrine tumours

Adjusted to the World-standard population the overall incidence was 2.39 per 100,000 inhabitants per year: 2.36 per 100,000 for women and 2.51 per 100,000 for men. Calculated to the US 2000 standard population the overall incidence was 2.99 per 100,000 inhabitants per year.

The age-specific incidence rate was highest between 50 and 70 years and began to increase at about 35 years.

Classification of the NETs according to the WHO criteria found that the overall incidence of tumours with benign, uncertain and malignant behaviour was 1.15, 0.43 and 0.81 per 100,000 inhabitants, respectively.

Age and sex of patients

Of the 285 patients, 148 were men and 137 women; their median ages at initial diagnosis were 63 (IQR: 22) and 59 (IQR: 27) years respectively (P value significant only before correction for multiple testing: P < 0.05, then non-significant). Patients with appendix NETs were significantly younger (median 38 [IQR: 45] years) than patients with NETs at any other site (P < 0.05).

Location

The site of the primary was the stomach in 65 (22.8%) patients, followed by the appendix (n = 59; 20.7%), the small intestine (excl. duodenum; n = 44; 15.4%), rectum (n = 40; 15.4%), pancreas (n = 33; 11.6%), colon (n = 20; 7.0%) and duodenum (n = 16; 5.6%). In one patient the tumour was located in the oesophagus, and in another patient in the gallbladder and Meckel's diverticulum (**Figure 3**; for analysis of the clinical data in Part 2 these three tumours were excluded).

Liver tumours expressing neuroendocrine markers were documented in five (1.7%) patients. By definition (see above), these tumours were categorized as metastasis from NETs located in various sites of the gastrointestinal tract. Adequate amounts of tissue were available for further immunohistochemical studies in three of the tumours: all three stained negative for serotonin. The definitive location of the primary remained unknown during the follow-up period of one year. These five tumours were excluded from further clinical analysis.

Differentiation and biological behaviour of neuroendocrine tumours

By definition [62], 131 (46.0%) NETs were classified as benign (incidence rate 1.15 per 100,000), 44 (15.4%) as having uncertain behaviour (incidence rate 0.43) and 110 (38.6%) as malignant (incidence rate 0.81). Among the malignant tumours 91 (82.7%; 31.9% of all 285 tumours) were well-differentiated and 19 (17.3%; 6.7% of all 285 tumours) were poorly differentiated.

Age/sex of patients and biological behaviour of tumours

The median age of patients with benign tumours was 60.0 (IQR: 26) years, with tumours of uncertain behaviour 51.0 (IQR: 37) years and with malignant tumours 65.5 (IQR: 18) years. Patients with benign or uncertain tumours were significantly younger than patients with malignant tumours (both P < 0.01); the ages of patients with benign and uncertain tumours were not significantly different from each other.

Even after excluding appendix NETs (patients with appendix NETs were significantly younger; 62.7% classified benign), patients with benign tumours were younger than patients with malignant tumours (P < 0.05) (uncertain vs. malignant and benign vs. uncertain: P not significant). Among patients with malignant tumours, the median age of those with well-differentiated tumours was 60.0 (IQR: 24) years and with poorly differentiated tumours 73.0 (IQR: 17) years (P < 0.05; after correction for multiple testing P not significant, 0.06).

The distribution of tumours with benign, uncertain and malignant behaviour was approximately equal in male and female patients for all tumour sites.

Location and biological behaviour of tumours

Whereas NETs of the stomach (67.7%), rectum (65%) and appendix (62.7%) were mainly classified as benign, those in the small intestine (86.4%), pancreas (75.8%) and colon (70.0%) were predominantly malignant (**Figure 1**).

Concerning tumour location, **Figure 4** summarizes the malignant NETs after subdividing them into well-differentiated and poorly differentiated. Four of five malignant rectal NETs were classified as poorly differentiated, whereas the proportions of this tumour type in all other sites except the duodenum were closely similar. Among PNETs, 20 (80.0%) of 25 were classified as well-differentiated and five as poorly differentiated endocrine carcinoma. Five of five malignant duodenal NETs were classified as well-differentiated.

Incidence of malignant NETs and other malignancies in the digestive tract

Table 1 summarizes the incidence of malignant NETs and all reported malignancies in the digestive tract. By definition, 1.49% of all malignant tumours of the digestive tract documented in the study period arose from neuroendocrine cells. In addition, 51.79% of all malignant tumours of the small intestine, 29.63% of all carcinomas of the appendix and 8.70% of duodenal malignancies were of neuroendocrine origin. The incidence of malignant gastrointestinal NETs was 0.81 per 100,000 inhabitants and the incidence of all reported malignancies in the digestive tract 54,49 per 100,000.

Distant metastasis

A total of 110 (38.6%) of 285 tumours were classified as malignant using the WHO criteria. At the time of diagnosis, information on metastasis was available in 87 (79.1%) patients. Lymph node or distant metastases were documented in 65 (74.7%) of 87 patients. The majority of distant metastases were located in the liver (n = 35: multiple 32, solitary 3), followed by the peritoneum (n = 11), bone (n = 4), lung (n = 2) ovary (n = 2) and brain (n = 1). Extended lymph node and distant metastases were documented in 29 (33.3%) patients.

TNM staging based on ENETS definitions

ENETS TNM classification and staging was possible in 181 (63.5%) of 277 tumours. Localised disease (lymph node negative) was documented in 118 (65.2%) of 181 tumours, regional disease (lymph node positive) in 20 (11.0%) and distant disease in 43 (23.8%), respectively. Applying the ENETS criteria, 74 tumours (46.4%) were stage I, 43 (23.8%) were stage II, 21 (11.6%) stage III and 43 (23.8%) stage IV independent of the location. Details are summarized in **Table 31**.

Histopathological grading based on ENETS criteria

Sufficient data were available in 77 (46.8%) of 277 tumours. The majority (46; 59.7%) of the tumours were grade 1, 24 (31.2%) were grade 2 and seven (9.1%) were grade 3. Of the seven tumours classified grade 3 one was located in the stomach, two in the pancreas, two in the colon and two in the rectum.

5.3.5 Discussion

This is the first study to analyse the incidence of GEP-NETs using a prospectively run data base. During a one-year period 285 tumours were recorded, resulting in an overall annual age-adjusted incidence rate (world standardized) of digestive NETs being 2.39 per 100,000 inhabitants per years. The results of the study, in which all locations of the digestive tract were included, show a higher incidence of GEP NETs than in other studies analysing similar populations [113, 114].

It may be assumed that nearly all newly diagnosed Austrian cases were recorded within the study period: 40 of 41 departments and institutes of clinical pathology, including four academic institutes, distributed throughout the country participated in the prospective study protocol and 31 institutes reported tumours diagnosed within the study period. This enables the analysis to attain a high degree of completeness. The numbers of patients diagnosed with GEP NETs, on the basis of standardized histopathological criteria, and the incidence of these tumours are therefore representative for a central European country with a highly developed medical training and social framework.

Because of sometimes vague clinical presentation and low awareness among physicians, data in the literature on the real incidence of NETs are probably underestimates. Data comparisons in relation to the site of tumour origin are difficult to obtain because of the overall rarity of these neoplasms and their incomplete recognition and documentation in various national cancer registries [115] and because of their variable and sometimes imprecise classification [103, 116].

NETs were not well-defined entities before 2000 [63] and national tumour databases offer population-based prospective documentation for malignant tumours only. The majority of these databases therefore under-report or even omit NETs classified as benign according to the WHO criteria [117, 118] and usually corresponding to grade 1 NETs according to the ENETS criteria [70].

Recently, Hauso et al. [107, 108] and Yao et al. [105] report a worldwide increasing incidence of NETs over the past three decades, suggesting that NETs are more prevalent than previously realised. These findings may partially reflect the more precise pathohistological definition of the neuroendocrine cells with the inclusion of those classified as benign in incidence studies. As shown in our study, NETs classified as benign are the largest group (46.0%). The higher incidence may also be associated with the incidental identification of small, asymptomatic lesions as the result of increased availability of endoscopic imaging of the upper and lower gastrointestinal tract and the broad use of early radiological imaging in addition to clinical examinations.

In discussion of the incidence of NETs, data from the SEER Program of the National Cancer Institute are usually cited [98, 107, 108]. The SEER registries may underestimate the total number of patients with NETs in various locations because all cases from the SEER database are by definition denoted to be malignant. It is therefore likely that small tumours with benign appearance may not generally be included in the SEER registries. One also has to keep in mind that all studies, including the SEER database, lack a standardized histopathological protocol for diagnosis.

In analysis of the late SEER period (1992–1999), Modlin et al. [98] presented incidence rates of 1.89 per 100,000 for white males and 1.59 per 100,000 for white females. Because of higher incidence rates in black males and females, the numbers for the white population may be best compared with European populations. More recently Hauso et al [107] compared the SEER NET data with the corresponding data of the Norwegian Registry of Cancer. The age-adjusted incidence rates extracted from 1993 to 2004 using as reference the US 2000 standard population for both databases calculated an incidence rate of 1.99 per 100,000 per year for Norway and of 2.3 for the USA (white subset of the SEER data; excluded lung/bronchus, urogenital tract, breast). The same calculation for Austria would show a higher incidence (2.99 per 100.000 per year; **Figure 5**) including all GEP NETs independent their presumed biological behaviour. This "statistical game" underlines the importance of adjusting incidence calculations to the same (and representative) "reference population".

Using the "World standard population" as reference Hemminki and Li [99] calculated incidence rates of 1.6 per 100,000 for males and 1.9 for females (no data for pancreas, liver or biliary tract) for Sweden (1983–1998). The incidence rates for Canton Vaud in Switzerland (1986–1997) given by Levi et al. [100] are 2.05 per 100,000 for males and 2.17 for females (no data for pancreas, liver or biliary tract) (**Figure 6**). The corresponding incidence data for Austria (World standard population; all gastro-entero-pancreatic sites) were 2.36 per 100,000 per year for female and 2.51 for males (**Figure 6**). In our prospective study more males than females had GEP NETs (1.08:1). This difference is more pronounced in the USA (1.2:1, [108]) and in Japan (2:1, [114]).

WHO classification – ENETS staging and grading

Using the WHO criteria[63], 175 (61.4%) tumours were classified as well-differentiated benign (131, 46.0%; WHO 1a) or uncertain (44, 15.4%; WHO 1b); a further 91 (31.9%) were well-differentiated (WHO 2) and 19 (6.7%) poorly differentiated (WHO 3) neuroendocrine carcinoma.

Using the ENETS staging criteria [70, 71], 40.9% of tumours were stage I and 23.8% stage II. ENETS stage III (IIIB) is defined as any T, (except location appendix) lymph node positive but distant metastasis negative and 11.0% fulfilled these criteria. In 23.8% stage IV was diagnosed, meaning that distant metastases were diagnosed at the time of initial diagnosis.

To our knowledge, the report by Levi et al. [100] is the only study distinguishing benign and malignant NETs on the basis of local infiltration and/or existence of metastasis: the incidence for benign NETs was 1.34 per 100,000 and for malignant tumours 0.72, the proportion of benign to malignant tumours being very similar to the data presented here (benign 1.15 per 100,000; uncertain 0.43; malignant 0.81).

Patients with malignant tumours were significantly older than patients with benign NETs, which raise the question of whether benign lesions transform into malignant tumours and therefore may be considered lesions with latent or low-grade malignancy. If this concept is accepted, the issue of early diagnosis and treatment becomes of critical clinical relevance.

In the present study 1.49% of all malignant digestive tumours were classified as NETs. GEP NETs are diagnosed less frequently than adenocarcinomas of the digestive tract. Among malignant tumours, GEP NETs constitute less than 2% of all gastrointestinal malignancies [119].

It has been widely discussed and long generally accepted that no histological grading system effectively predicts the behaviour of well-differentiated endocrine tumours [70]. However, a grading system has been introduced by ENETS [70, 71] partly adopting the WHO criteria. In our study, G3 tumours were diagnosed only in the stomach, colon, rectum and pancreas.

Location

Stomach

The present study reveals the stomach as the preferential location (22.8% of all GEP NETs) as suspected by Klöppel and colleagues [77, 120]. This is in contrast to other studies [98, 113, 121, 122] describing NETs of the small intestine most frequently. Reviewing clinical single-centre studies, gastric NETs are recorded as 3.1% to 13.8% [123]. NETs of the stomach comprised 4.1% of all gastrointestinal NETs in the late SEER [98] and 8% in the population-based study from western Norway [113]. An explanation for the increase may be the large number and liberal use of endoscopic diagnostic procedures, with biopsies routinely taken from all, even small, gastric lesions.

By definition [62], 67.7% of the gastric lesions in our study were classified as NETs with benign behaviour, 12.3% as uncertain and 20.0% as malignant. The incidence of malignant NETs in the stomach was low, calculated as 0.08 per 100,000. In contrast to other studies [124], a higher proportion of benign tumours in women with stomach NETs was not documented in our study.

Duodenum/small intestine

Even when small intestine (15.4%) and duodenal (5.6%) NETs are added together (21.0%), the stomach remains the most frequent location in our study. Previously, duodenal NETs accounted for 3.8% of all gastrointestinal NETs and were integrated in the group of small-bowel NETs in older series (total 25.2%) [98]. It appears unjustified to sum NETs of the small intestine and duodenum since our data document that small-intestine NETs are predominantly malignant (86.4%) and duodenal NETs are more often benign (62.5%). The incidence of malignant NETs in the duodenum was very low at 0.02 per 100,000 whereas the incidence of malignant NETs in the ileum/jejunum was 0.29 per 100,000.

Pancreas

In our study the overall annual incidence of PNETs was 0.25 per 100,000, subdividing into benign, uncertain and malignant at 0.02, 0.04 and 0.19 per 100,000 respectively. The annual incidence of PNETs was reviewed recently and was described as < 0.4 cases per 100,000 [125], accounting for only 1–3% of all pancreatic neoplasms.

Appendix

Patients with appendiceal NETs were significantly younger (median 38.0 years) than patients with tumours at all other sites: children and adults ≤ 20 years may be affected, as found in five (8.9%) of 56 patients. One may speculate that appendiceal NETs are diagnosed incidentally during appendectomy because appendicitis is diagnosed more often in younger patients. Overall, appendiceal NETs accounted for 20.7% of all gastrointestinal NETs, the majority (62.7%) being classified as benign, 27.1% as uncertain and 10.2% as malignant. The incidence of malignant NETs in this location was 0.08 per 100,000 population. Although the frequency of appendiceal NETs has decreased over time [98], NETs are the most frequent type of tumour in the appendix and can be expected in 1 of 200 appendectomies [97]. They rarely reach clinical significance.

Colon and rectum

In the analysis by Modlin et al., 1481 (21.2%) of 6996 digestive NETs were localised in the rectum, comprising 1–2% of all rectal tumours, and 938 (21.2%) were in the colon [98, 126]. In the current study, 40 (14%) of 285 GEP NETs were located in the rectum and 20 (7%) in the colon. Although the majority of those in the rectum were classified as benign (26 of 40, 65%), the incidence of malignant rectal NETs being only 0.03 per 100,000 population, 14 (70%) of 20 colonic NETs were classified as neuroendocrine carcinoma (well-differentiated 10, 71%; poorly differentiated 4, 29%; 0.13 per 100,000).

Conclusion

Standard cancer registries do not reflect the real incidence, because benign tumours are omitted from many national registries. Using strict pathohistological/ immunohistochemical criteria the incidence of benign and malignant gastrointestinal NETs has been demonstrated for the first time in a middle European country. As presumed, NETs are most frequently located in the stomach followed by the sites appendix, small intestine, rectum, pancreas and colon. Subdividing them into groups as recommended by the WHO, 46% of NETs were classified as "benign", 15% as showing "uncertain" biological behaviour and 39% as showing "malignant" behaviour. Using the ENETS TNM classification a minority of gastrointestinal NETs were classified as Stage IIIB (N positive 11.0%; regional disease) and IV (N and/or M positive 23.8%; distant disease) at the time of diagnosis. In the ENETS grading the majority of NETs were G1 (59.7%) and G2 (31.2%) independent of their staging. G3 tumours are very rare (9.1%).

Declaration of interest: There is no conflict of interest that could be perceived as prejudicing the impartiality of the research reported.

Funding: This research did not receive any specific grant from any funding agency in the public, commercial or not-for-profit sector.

Author contributions: This manuscript is part of M.B. Niederle's doctoral thesis 'Neuroendocrine tumours of the digestive tract in Austria' (N090 Endocrinology and Metabolism), for obtaining the academic title Doctor of Medical Science at the Medical University of Vienna.

Acknowledgements: The authors wish to thank Bettina Haidbauer for running the study secretariat and the members of the Austrian Society of Clinical Pathology for supporting this national study.

5.3.6 Tables and Figures

Site	Incidence in digestive tract (per 100,000 population)		Digestive malignant NETs: percentage of all malignancies
	Malignant NETs*	All reported malignancies**	
Oesophagus	0.01	2,55	0,39
Stomach	0.08	8,16	0,98
Duodenum	0.02	0,23	8,70
Pancreas	0.19	8,31	2,29
Small intestine excl. duodenum	0.29	0,56	51,79
Appendix	0.08	0,27	29,63
Colon (incl. rectosigmoid junction)	0.06	18,19	0,33
Rectum	0.03	9,73	0,31
Liver	0.05	5,48	0,91
Meckel diverticulum	0.00	0,01	0,00
Gall bladder incl. bile duct	0.00	1,00	0,00
Total	0.81	54,49	1,49

Table 30 - Site and incidence of malignant neuroendocrine tumours and other malignancies of the digestive tract

Stage		T	N	M	Stomach	Duodenum/ Ampulla	Pancreas	Prox/dist Jejunum/ Ileum	Appendix	Colon	Rectum	Total
n					65	16	33	44	59	20	40	277
n*					35 [8m]	7 [2m]	29	31	48	10	21	181/277 (65.3%)
		X										
		Tis										
I	IA	1 / 1a**	0	0	25 (71.4%)	3 (42.9%)	5 (17.2%)	2 (6.5%)	19 (39.6%)	1 (10%)	13 (61.9%)	74/181 (40.9%)
	IB	1b***	0	0	1 (2.9%)	2 (28.6%)	6 (20.7%)	1 (3.2%)	18 (37.5%)	2 (20%)	4 (19.0%)	
II	IIA	2	0	0	2 (5.7%)	0	2 (6.9%)	2 (6.5%)	8 (16.7%)	0	1 (4.8%)	43/181 (23.8%)
	IIB	3	0	0	0	0	0	0	1 (2.1%)	0	0	
III	IIIA	4	0	0	1 (2.9%)	0	3 (10.3%)	11 (35.5%)	1 (2.1%)	3 (30%)	1 (4.8%)	21/181 (11.6%)
	IIIB	anyT	1	0								
IV	IV	anyT	anyN	1	6 (17.1%)	2 (28.6%)	13 (44.8%)	15 (48.4%)	1 (2.1%)	4 (40%)	2 (9.5%)	43/181 (23.8%)

* n patients with ENETS TNM classification/staging
TX: Primary tumour could not be assessed, T0: No evidence of primary tumour; Tis: In situ tumour/dysplasia (<0.5cm) – stomach; For any T add (m) for multiple tumours
** T1a and *** T1b: Colon/rectum – tumour invades mucosa or submucosa T1a size <1 cm; T1b size 1–2 cm
NX: Regional lymph node status could not be assessed; N0: No regional lymph node metastasis; N1: Regional lymph node metastasis
MX: Distant metastasis could not be assessed; M0: No distant metastases; M1: Distant metastasis

Table 31 - ENETS staging based on details of 181 of 277 (65.3%) patients

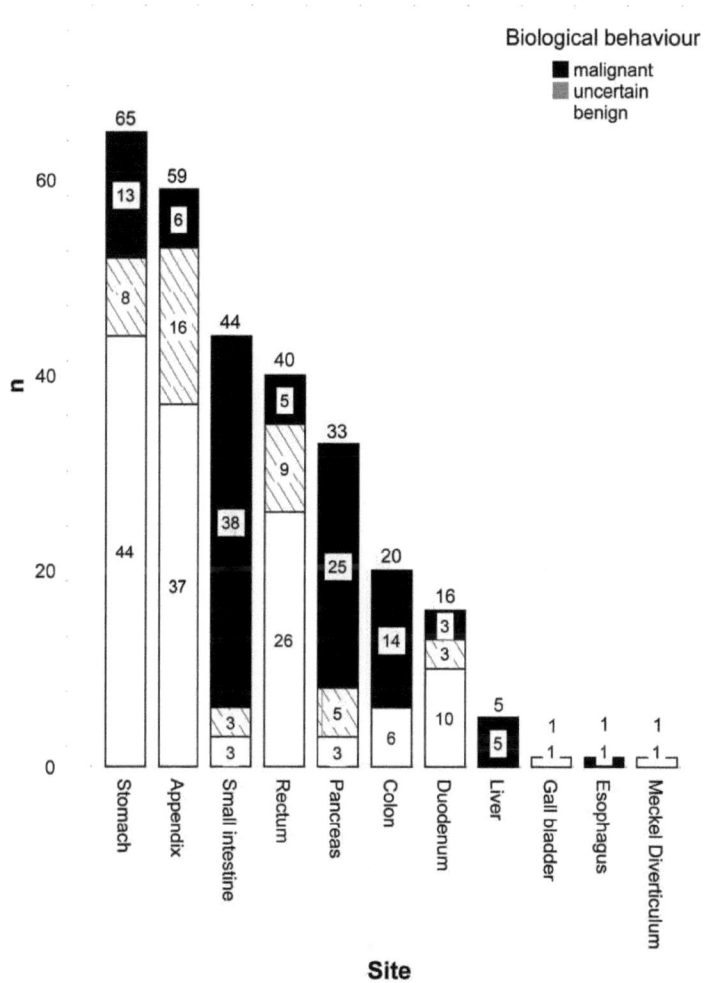

Figure 3 - Number (%), location and biological behaviour of neuroendocrine tumours in each site

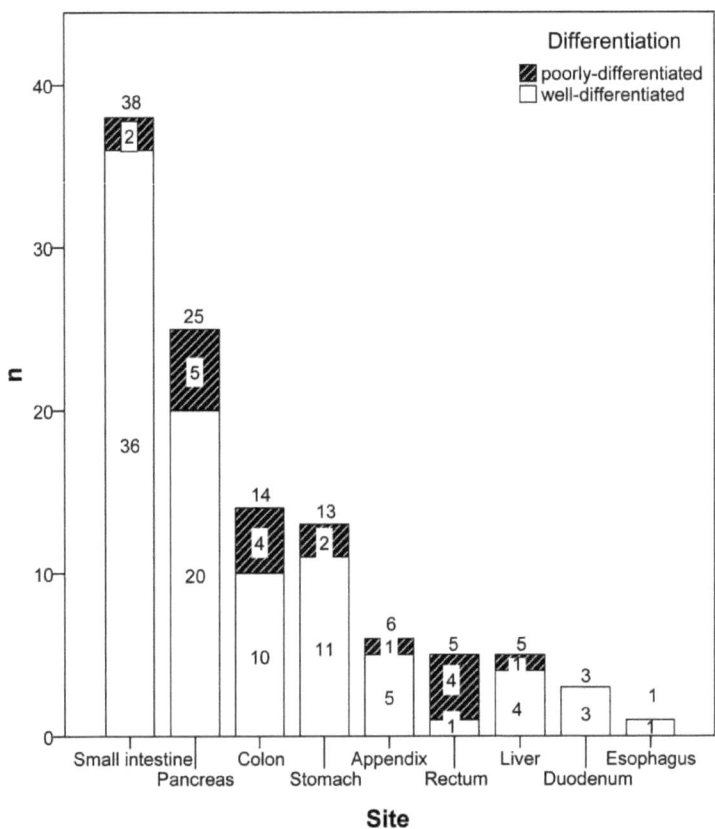

Figure 4 - Malignant neuroendocrine tumours of the digestive tract – well-differentiated and poorly-differentiated neuroendocrine carcinoma

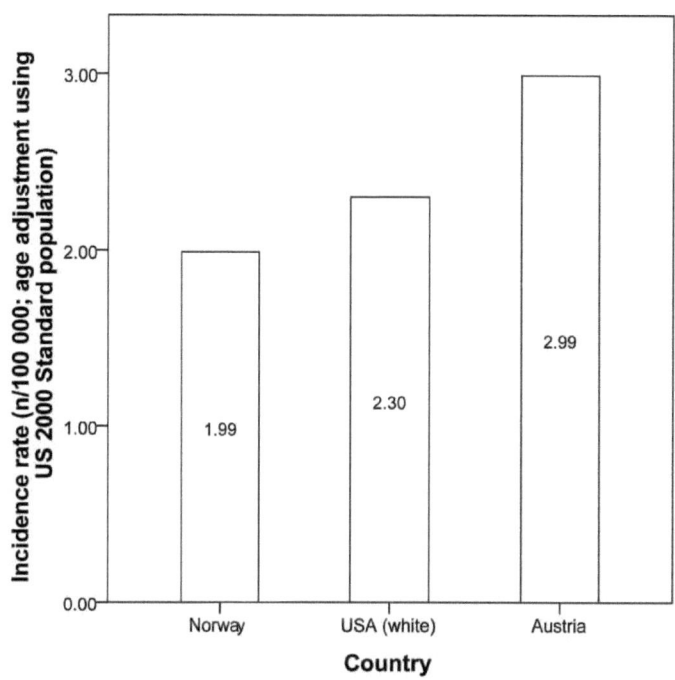

Figure 5 - Incidence rates of GEP neuroendocrine tumours (n/100,000/year); age-adjusted using the US 2000 standard population comparing the recent data with Norway and the USA [107]

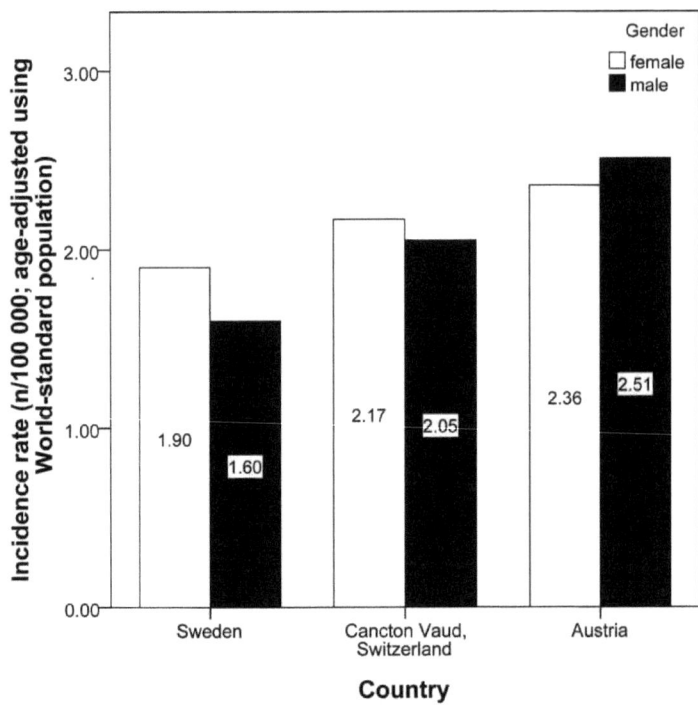

Figure 6 - Incidence rates of GEP neuroendocrine tumours (n/100,000/year); age-adjusted using the world standard population comparing the recent data with Sweden [99] and Switzerland [100]

5.4 Diagnosis and treatment of gastroenteropancreatic neuroendocrine tumours - Current data on a prospectively collected, retrospectively analyzed clinical multicenter investigation

Original paper 2 published in
Oncologist 2011; 16(5):602-13 doi: 10.1634/theoncologist.2011-0002
Authors: Martin B. Niederle, M.D. and Bruno Niederle, M.D.

Short title: Diagnosis and treatment of GEP-NETs

Synopsis: Clinical information concerning diagnosis, symptoms and treatment of 277 patients with gastrointestinal neuroendocrine tumors (incl. pancreas) diagnosed prospectively within one year were analyzed. Endoscopic and surgical techniques are the key to both correct diagnosis and effective treatment.

Keywords: neuroendocrine tumors – gastrointestinal tract – diagnosis and treatment – prospective clinical trial

5.4.1 Abstract

Background. The aim of this prospectively collected, retrospectively analyzed clinical investigation was to describe "unmasked" clinical symptoms, method of diagnosis, treatment, and short-term follow-up of gastroenteropancreatic-neuroendocrine tumors (GEP-NETs) diagnosed during one year in Austria.

Methods. In total 277 patients with GEP-NETs were documented. All tumors were immunhistochemically defined according to recently summarized criteria (WHO, ENETS). A standardized questionnaire comprising 50 clinical and biochemical parameters (clinical symptoms, mode-of-diagnosis, treatment, follow-up) was completed by attending physicians.

Results. The most common initial symptoms were episodes of abdominal-pain, diarrhea, weight-loss, gastrointestinal-bleeding, flushing, and bowel-obstruction. Overall 48.1% of tumors were diagnosed by endoscopy, 43.7% during surgery, 5% by fine-needle aspiration of the primary or metastases, and 2.5% during autopsy;

44.5% of tumors were not suspected clinically and were diagnosed incidentally during various surgical procedures. Overall 18.7% were removed endoscopically and 67.6% surgically; 13.7% were followed without interventional treatment. Endoscopic/surgical intervention was curative in 81.4% of patients, palliative in 18.6%. At the time of diagnosis, information on metastasis was available in 83.7% with malignant NETs. Lymph node or distant metastases were documented in 74.7%. In 34/176 (19.3%) patients 41 secondary tumors were documented, 78.0% being classified histologically as adenocarcinomas. During a 1-year follow-up 61.5% showed no evidence of disease, 13.5% had stable disease, 16.7% showed progression of disease, and in 8.3% the NET was the cause of death.

Conclusion. This investigation summarizes the clinical presentation and current practice of management of GEP-NETs and thereby extends the understanding and clinical experience.

5.4.2 Introduction

NETs are a heterogeneous group arising from neuroendocrine cells and show distinct functional and biological behavior depending on location, tumor size and clinical symptoms [62]. Correct pathohistological diagnosis is the key to adequate treatment [103] and it is crucial to classify lesions as NETs only if they stain immunohistochemically positive for chromogranin A and/or synaptophysin [103].

Although some NETs behave benign, all are potentially malignant [62]. In a prospectively designed incidence study [127], 46% of NETs were classified as "well-differentiated benign" (WHO 2000 1a), 43% as "well-differentiated benign/low-grade malignant with uncertain biological behavior" (WHO 2000 1b), and 39% as showing malignant behavior (WHO 2000 2: well-differentiated/low-grade malignant carcinoma; WHO 2000 3: poorly differentiated/high-grade malignant carcinoma) [63, 127]. Using the TNM classification proposed by the European Neuroendocrine Tumour Society (ENETS) [70, 71], 11.0% were classified as stage III (lymph-node positive; regional disease) and 23.8% stage IV (M positive; distant disease) [127]. Poorly differentiated (Grade 3) tumors were found in 9.1% [127].

The aim of the present prospectively collected, retrospectively analyzed clinical investigation was to describe "unmasked" clinical symptoms, diagnostic procedures, treatment, and short-term follow-up of precisely classified GEP-NETs. This approach documenting "everyday routine" should extend the knowledge and clinical experience of this rare tumor entity and should add cornerstones for earlier diagnosis and application of the guidelines on the treatment, thereby improving the clinical outcome. Furthermore the risk stratification comparing the WHO 2000 and the new WHO 2010 classifications should be demonstrated.

5.4.3 Methods

Background of the clinical investigation

In a previous prospective trial to clarify the incidence of GEP-NETs in Austria, consecutive tumors histologically/immunhistochemically diagnosed and classified as NETs were documented in 285 patients during a 1-year period (May 1, 2004 to April 30, 2005) [127].

The site of the primary was the stomach in 65 (22.8%) patients, followed by the appendix (n = 59; 20.7%), small intestine excluding duodenum (n = 44; 15.4%), rectum (n = 40; 15.4%), pancreas (n = 33; 11.6%), colon (n = 20; 7.0%), and duodenum (n = 16; 5.6%) [127].

In one patient each the tumor was located in the esophagus, gallbladder, and Meckel diverticulum; liver tumors expressing neuroendocrine markers were documented in five (1.7%) patients. These eight tumors were categorized as metastasis from NETs located in various sites of the gastrointestinal tract [103], the location of the primary remaining unknown during the follow-up period. These eight patients were excluded from further analysis, thus 277 (97.2%) patients generated the background of the detailed clinical analysis.

In the former study [127] 277 tumors were classified according to WHO 2000 [62, 63]. 77 (27.9%) were graded according to ENETS 2006/2007 [70, 71]. Therefore a reclassification according WHO 2010 [69] and, as an example, a comparison of both classifications were performed.

In addition to the pathological report [127], details on the natural clinical course of the disease were requested in questionnaires comprising 50 clinical and biochemical parameters (clinical reports). The attending physicians were invited to participate in the multicenter study.

Informed consent

All patients were asked for informed consent for their clinical data to be documented. The full names of the patients remained unknown to the study center.

Analysis and presentation of clinical data

Patients were integrated into the clinical database only if they had agreed to participate in the study, thus some could not be included. In addition, some questionnaires were incompletely filled out lacking basic information. As a minimum requirement, information on the presence of metastasis (present/absent) and/or treatment had to be available for integration of a patient's data into the database. All available clinical parameters were included in a Filemaker® database (clinical database) and analyzed using SPSS® Version 17.0 (Chicago, Illinois, USA).

The clinical data are summarzied in the tables **Table 33-38**. Because some questionnaires were returned incomplete (missing parameters for some patients) the tables also include the description, how often certain information were "available" or "unavailable" (missing information) to present data in a correct and objective manner ("data quality").

Ethics committee resolution

The prospective study design, manner of data collection, and the retrospective analysis were approved by the ethics committee of the Medical University of Vienna (Resolution number 157/2005).

5.4.4 Results

WHO 2000 versus WHO 2010

According to the WHO 2000 [62, 63] 46 (59.7%) of 77 NETS in various locations were classified "well differentiated endocrine tumors" ("benigne" – WHO 1a: 33 [42.9%]; "uncertain" - WHO 1b: 13 [16.9%]), 24 (31.2%) as "well differentiated endocrine carcinoma" and 7 (9.1%) as "poorly differentiated endocrine carcinoma" (**Table 32**). According to the proposal of the current WHO 2010 classification [69] 46 (59.7%) of 77 tumors were reclassified as "NET G1 (carcinoid)", 24 (31.2%) as "NET G2" and 7 (9.1%) as "neuroendocrine carcinoma" respectively (**Table 32**).

Clinical symptoms, method of diagnosis, biochemical data

The most *common symptoms* among 241 (87.0%) of the 277 patients analyzed were abdominal pain (71/241; 29.5%), diarrhea (21/241; 8.7%), weight loss (18/241; 7.5%), gastrointestinal bleeding (13/241; 5.4%), flushing (9/241; 3.7%), and bowel obstruction (8/241; 3.3%). Neurological and psychiatric symptoms were reported in 5 (2.1%) patients, among whom were 3/33 (9.1%) patients with pancreatic NETs. In two of the three patients insulinomas may have been suspected clinically but were not confirmed biochemically because no specific functional tests were performed; an insulinoma was documented biochemically in the third patient. Diarrhea was the leading clinical symptom in one biochemically confirmed VIPoma. One other patient suffered from recurrent peptic ulcers. Gastrinoma may have been suspected clinically but was not confirmed biochemically because no "secretin tests" were applied.

The majority of tumors were *diagnosed* in departments of surgery (180/277 [64.9%]) followed by departments of internal medicine (90/277 [32.5%]). Seven tumours (pancreas n=5; small intestine: 2; [2.5%]) not suspected clinically as NETS were finally documented during autopsy.

As shown in **Table 33**, 135 (48.1%) of 277 tumours were diagnosed by endoscopy, 121 (43.7%) during surgery (see also "incidental diagnosis), 4 (1.4%) by fine needle aspiration of the primary and 10 (3.6 %) of metastases, respectively.

Biochemical data were available in 34 (12.3%) of the 277 analyzed patients. Specific laboratory tests (gastrin, insulin, C peptide, VIP, serotonin, 5-hydroxindole acetic acid, chromogranin A) were not used routinely. Elevated levels of gastrin were documented in all five (WHO 1a) tumors of the stomach and in the two (WHO 1a) tumors of the duodenum. Elevated hormone levels indicating functioning pancreatic NETs were documented in two patients: insulinoma (positive 48h-fast-test) and VIPoma in one patient each. Elevated levels of 5-hydroxindole acetic acid were documented in the urine (carcinoid syndrome) of 2/9 (22.2%) patients with tumors of the small intestine and liver metastases. One pancreatic NET was associated with multiple endocrine neoplasia 1 (MEN1) syndrome (1/112; 0.9%).

Treatment

A total of 147 (67.1%) tumors were treated surgically and 41 (18.7%) endoscopically; 30 (13.7%) lesions were followed without interventional treatment (**Table 34**). As preparation for treatment of liver metastasis, one patient (0.5%) underwent cholecystectomy without treating the NET. Overall, details of interventions were documented in 188/277 patients (67.9%) (**Table 35**).

Stomach

Of 35 stomach tumors, 20 (57.1%) were removed endoscopically and 15 (42.9%) surgically (**Table 33**). Stepwise biopsy of the gastric mucosa was performed in 38/65 (58.5%) patients. Details on the association of chronic atrophic gastritis type A (CAG) were available in 38 (58.5%) patients; CAG was described in 32 (84.2%). Three NETs (all WHO 2000: 1a) were diagnosed concomitantly with an adenocarcinoma of the stomach.

Endoscopic mucosectomy or polypectomy and subtotal or total gastrectomy were performed (**Table 35**). In three lesions classified as WHO 2000: 1a/ENETS T1N0M0, the indication for subtotal (n = 1) or total gastrectomy (n = 2) was the NET (**Table 35**).

Duodeum

Nine (81.9%) of 11 tumors were removed endoscopically, 5 (45.5%) surgically (**Table 35**).

Pancreas

13 (50.0%) of 26 pancreatic tumours were localised in the pancreatic head, 7 (26.9%) in the pancreatic body and 6 (23.1%) in the pancreatic tail.

Left pancreatic resection was performed in 7/20 (35.0%) patients, Whipple operation in 5 (25.0%), tumor enucleation in 5 (25.0%), central pancreatic resection in 1 (5.0%), tumor debulking in 1 (5.0%), and gastroenterostomy in 1 (5.0%).

Small intestine

Among 44 patients, 28 (63.3%) were treated surgically. Small intestine segment resection, right hemicolectomy, and ileocecal resection were performed. One patient underwent cholecystectomy without treatment of the NET.

Appendix

In 45 (88.2%) of 51 patients the tumour was located at the tip, in 6 (11.8%) near or at the base of the appendix.

Interventions were documented in 56/59 (94.9%) patients: 47 (83.9%) had one surgical intervention, 9 (16.1%) had re-operations after initial appendectomy (**Table 34**). During re-operations hemicolectomy was performed in 7 patients, ileocecal resection and local lymphadenectomy in one patient each (**Table 34**).

Colon

Of 15 colonic tumors, 11 (73.3%) were removed surgically and 4 (26.7%) endoscopically. Hemicolectomy, endoscopic polypectomy, subtotal colectomy, and sigma resection were performed. In two cases, both classified as WHO 1a/T1N0M0, the indication for hemicolectomy/sigma resection was the NET.

Rectum

Details on therapeutic procedures were available in 29/40 (72.5%) tumors: 13 (44.8%) were removed surgically, 13 (44.8%) endoscopically. Endoscopical polypectomy, anterior rectal resection, and transanal resection (mucosectomy) were performed. In two patients the indication for anterior rectal resection was the NET.

Overall, 105/129 (81.4%) surgical interventions were intended to be curative, 24 (18.6%) palliative.

Distant metastasis

At the time of diagnosis information concerning metastasis was available in 87 (83.7%) of 104 patients with malignant NETs (**Table 36**). 65 of 87 (74.7%) tumors had already metastasized. Small intestinal malignant NETs had metastasis in 27 (87.1%) of 31 patients. 45 (51.7%) patients had metastasis in lymph nodes and 35 (40.2%) in the liver. Both, lymph node and distant metastases were documented in 29 (33.3%) of 87 patients.

Additional malignancy

Of the 277 patients analyzed, clinical data on additional malignancies were available in 176 (61.7%). Forty-one various tumors, their location, and the time of diagnosis are described in Table 4. Among these, 32 (78.0%) were classified histologically as adenocarcinomas: 19 (46.3%) localized in the colon or rectum, 7 in the urogenital tract, 6 (14.6%) in the breast (**Table 37**). Six of seven adenocarcinomas of the stomach were associated with NETs of the stomach and CAG.

Medical treatment
Data were available for 70/104 (67.3%) malignant tumors. Forty (57.1%) patients did not receive medical treatment. Somatostatin analogs were used in 20/27 (74.1%) patients, interferon in 7/23 (30.4%), and chemotherapy in 10/22 (45.5%).
Various treatment modalities were reported for 18/35 (51.4%) patients with liver metastases: ablation chemoembolization in 10 (55.6%), selective internal radiotherapy in 4 (22.2%), radio-frequency ablation in 1 (5.6%). Peptide receptor radiotherapy was used in 3/17 (16.7%). (see **Table 38**)

Follow-up
One year after diagnosis, follow-up data were documented in 96 (34.7%) of the 277 analyzed patients: 59 (61.5%) showed no evidence of disease, 13 (13.5%) had stable disease, 16 (16.7%) had progression of disease, and 8 (8.3%) died as the result of the NET. The patients with disease progression developed local recurrence in 9 (9.4%) cases and new distant metastases in 15 (15.6%).

5.4.5 Discussion

This analysis documents the clinical management of 277 consecutive GEP-NETs precisely classified as NETs [103] and grouped according to the WHO 2000 [62, 63]. Additionally in 181 (65.3%) patients the ENETS staging [70, 71] and in 77 (27.9%) the ENETS grading [70, 71] were applied.

The WHO 2000 classification [62, 63] in combination with the ENETS TNM classification and grading system [70, 71], served as a basis for establishing criteria for practical management especially in Europe [24]. Because of a low acceptance of both systems in the USA, the WHO developed a revised version for the classification of NETs. Taking all European and American arguments into account the WHO 2010 [69] classification consists of a grading system which is combined with a site-specific staging system (identical with the AJCC/UICC-TNM-System [details see: [69]). WHO 2010 eliminates the clinically inefficient group of patients with tumors of "uncertain behaviour" [128]. Based on the consideration that all NETS are malignant but may behave differently based on their specific grading [69], there were in fact minor changes in the "risk stratification" comparing WHO 2000 and WHO 2010. In detail 53.8% of WHO 2000 Type1b tumors ("uncertain clinical behaviour") shifted to

"Neuroendocrine Tumors G1" and 46.2% to "Neuroendocrine Tumors G2" and are now better risk-stratified.

Because reclassification was impossible for all patients and because of the limited experience with the WHO 2010 classification, the combination of the WHO 2000 [62, 63] and the ENETS grading and staging system [70, 71] was used for presenting and discussing this clinical investigation. Since there are only marginal differences between the combination of WHO 2000 [62, 63] and ENETs grading and staging system [70, 71] compared to the new WHO 2010 classification, the conclusions are valid for both the old and the new classifications.

The predominant part of the tumors was diagnosed using endoscopic techniques (48.1%). This high percentage is mainly due to the fact, that particular lesions in the stomach (96.9%), the rectum (90.0%), the duodenum (81.2%) and the colon (55.0%) were detected during endoscopy. Most of these tumors were small, benign and incidental findings.

Unsuspected clinically as NETs, 43.7% were found during surgery, mainly located in the appendix (98.3%), the small intestine (63.6%), the pancreas (51.5%) and the colon (45.0%). Only a minority was detected by fine-needle aspiration biopsy (FNA) of the tumor itself (1.4%) or of a (liver-)metastasis (3.6%).

Nonspecific symptoms (vague abdominal pain, weight loss) were evident in 37%. Retrospectively, specific clinical symptoms either local (e.g. local stenosis, melena) or systemic (e.g. diarrhea, flushing) were reported in 21.5%. This is in accordance with earlier and current experience [129]. Landerholm et al. [130] reported that even small bowel NETs with distant metastasis may present without symptoms and the carcinoid syndrome is infrequently seen. Aggarwal et al. [131] therefore recommended that primary-care physicians should keep in mind NETs and their vague, nonspecific clinical features and start appropriate diagnostic testing early.

Only a small group of patients (12.3%) underwent comprehensive endocrine testing to confirm the functionality of the NETs. However, the absence of documented functionality does not exclude a hormonally active syndrome in many patients. On reviewing single-center reports from referral centers [132] and recently established national registries [121, 133], functioning tumors were reported in up to 40% of patients. Up to 49% localized in the small intestine [88, 121, 134] and up to 75% in the pancreas [125, 128] were functioning. In our study, the lack of more patients with functioning tumors and endocrine tumor syndromes in various sites (pancreas, ileum/jejunum) is surprising but reflects the "general" situation. Although clinical data were collected prospectively, it is not possible to determine whether indeed pancreatic NETs are mainly non-functioning or whether functioning tumors and tumor syndromes were not documented as such. Nevertheless, the low reporting of typical symptoms of hormonal activity may indicate a greater proportion of non-functioning tumors than previously assumed. The higher rates of functioning tumors in larger, mainly academic series may reflect a single-center effect [133].

More and more NETs in the upper and lower gastrointestinal tract are treated successfully by various endoscopic techniques. Candidate tumors for endoscopic resection are localized and well-differentiated with very low risk of metastasis [103]. Endoscopic excision of various tumors was performed in 18.6%.

Typical surgical resections (with/without lymph node dissection) were performed in 67.8%. The domain for radical surgical intervention (with/without additional treatment) is that of NETs localized in the pancreas, ileum/jejunum, and appendix, and in more advanced tumors in all locations with the intention of curative resection (ENETS stage 3; [103]). Palliative surgery may be considered in selected patients with well-differentiated low-grade carcinoma (ENETS stage 4) [103].

In the majority (81.4%) of patients the surgical procedure was curative (R0). The high rate of curative procedures was influenced by the number of NETs localized in the appendix and classified as "benign" or "uncertain". As an alternative to endoscopic or surgical treatment, medical treatment (somatostatin analogs, interferon, chemotherapy, or combinations of various regimens) was offered to 42.9% including patients with very advanced malignant disease. It is recommended that fast-growing, poorly differentiated tumors (WHO 2000:3; WHO 2010: neuroendocrine carcinoma) of all T classifications, with lymph node and/or distant metastases, are initially treated by chemotherapy [103].

Overall, distant metastases were demonstrated in 74.7% of all malignant NETs. Because 51.7% of all patients with malignant tumors had metastasis in lymph nodes a radical approach with lymph node dissection seems mandatory in surgical treatment. 40.2% of all malignant tumors had metastasized to the liver It is well-recognized that at the time of initial diagnosis multiple liver metastases may be present even though the primary localized in the digestive tract may be clinically silent [129].

According to the ENETS grading [70, 71] and corresponding to the WHO 2010 [69] G3 tumors were diagnosed only in the colon, rectum, and pancreas. Although lymph node (35.5%) and distant metastases (48.4%) are diagnosed very early in the clinical course of ileum/jejunum NETs, all were graded G1 and G2, indicating an overall good prognosis. In the series reported by Landersholm et al. [130] metastasized tumors (44% regional; 40% distant) were classified as WHO 2000: 2.

Clinical presentation, tumor aggressiveness and metastatic potential, and the prognosis depend upon the primary location [135]

Stomach

According to the WHO [62], gastric NETs, heading the list of GEP-NETs [127], are classified into four biologically distinct types [120, 136]. Correct diagnosis and adequate treatment are based on precise classification and risk stratification [103]. However, in our study not all 65 gastric NETs could be subdivided into types 1, 2, 3 or 4 according to the underlying pathophysiological stimulus [137] and morphology [120]. Gastrin levels were determined in only 8 (12%) patients and hypergastrinemia was documented in five patients with WHO 2000: 1a tumors. Type 1 tumors may be suspected indirectly in 32/38 (84%) patients because CAG Type A was documented histologically after stepwise biopsy of the gastric mucosa [138].

In accordance with the ENETS guidelines [64, 78], endoscopic polypectomy or mucosectomy was documented in 20/35 (57.1%) patients. This appears adequate for 19 of the 20 patients; one patient underwent mucosectomy for a NET classified as well-differentiated malignant. Two patients with adenocarcinoma of the stomach underwent subtotal gastrectomy, the NETs (WHO 2000: 1a) being diagnosed synchronously. Gastrectomy was performed in 10 patients; overtreatment may be discussed in three patients with sole WHO 2000: 1a and 1b lesions.

Duodenum

Small duodenal tumors may be locally resected by endoscopy or surgery [64], as performed in six of nine patients. One well-differentiated carcinoma in the duodenal bulb was removed by distal gastric resection, one by pancreatic head resection [64].

Pancreas

Functioning PNETs may be suspected in only 5/33 (15.1%) patients. Biochemical parameters confirmed insulinoma and VIPoma in one patient each. Depending on the function, size, and location in the pancreas [103, 128], enucleation or major resections (with lymph node dissection for diagnostic and therapeutic purposes) were performed in 5 and 15 patients, respectively.

Jejunum/ileum

Curative surgery is always recommended whenever feasible after careful symptomatic control of the clinical syndrome with somatostatin analogs [88]. Surgery of the primary should be performed as segmental resection, ileocecal resection, or right hemicolectomy with wide lymphadenectomy depending on the localization of the tumor [88]. These procedures were performed in 13 (46.6%), 7 (25%), and 7 (25%) of 28 patients. Curative surgery was achieved in 16/26 (61.5%) patients.

Appendix

NETs in the appendix rarely reach clinical significance. Apart from one patient (1.7%), all tumors (98.3%) were incidentally diagnosed histologically after appendectomy. Clinically, acute appendicitis was the indication for simple appendectomy in 89.2%. Forty-seven (83.9%) of 56 patients had one surgical intervention. Re-operations were performed in 9 (16.1%) patients: hemicolectomy in 7, ileocecal resection in 1, local lymphadenectomy in 1. According to the ENETS guidelines [90, 139], the indication and extent of re-operation was justified in at least 8 (88.9%) of these 9 patients.

Colon and rectum

NETs of the colon should be treated in a similar way to adenocarcinoma of the colon, with localized colectomy and radical lymphadenectomy [91]. This concept was used in 11/15 (73.3%) patients. The treatment of WHO 1a and 1b rectal NETs includes endoscopic polypectomy, transanal excision (mucosectomy), or extended resection [91, 140]. Minimally invasive techniques are safe and were performed in 21/26 (80.8%) NETs. The extent of surgery seems not justified in the two patients with well-differentiated benign tumors and in the patient with poorly differentiated endocrine carcinoma. The poor prognosis of the latter is due to frequent presentation with metastases at the time of first diagnosis and the relative lack of effective therapy [89]. Selected patients with regional disease (N0/1 M0) may benefit from surgery whereas those with distant disease (M1) are best treated initially with chemotherapy.

Additional malignancy

Patients with GEP-NETs have an up to 46% risk of synchronous or metachronous neoplasia in various locations [141-143]. Thus, forty-one malignant tumors were documented synchronously, before or after the diagnosis of the GEP-NET in 34/176 (19.3%) patients. Among these tumors, 19 (46.3%) were adenocarcinoma localized in the stomach, colon, or rectum. NETs in the rectum (24%) and colon (23.1%) had the highest rate of secondary primary malignancies, followed by NETs in the stomach (19.0%), appendix (18.6%), jejunum/ileum (18.0%), and pancreas (8.9%). This is in contrast to analysis reporting small intestine NETs as having the highest rate of secondary primary malignancies, followed by appendiceal and colorectal NETs [123]. Among the additional malignancies, 21/41 (51.2%) were diagnosed synchronously and 14 (34.1%) before the diagnosis of the NET. However, 6 (14.6%) secondary carcinomas were diagnosed within the first year after NET diagnosis. In contrast to the conclusion of Brune et al. [144], long-term follow-up is recommended for patients with NETs, for both secondary malignancies and delayed metastasis.

Follow-up

The follow-up time of one year is too short to analyze the overall survival and calculate the prognosis. However, after one year 75.0% of the patients showed no evidence of disease or had stable disease, 16.7% showed progression, and in 8.3%

the NET was the cause of death. Only patients with tumors classified as well-differentiated or poorly differentiated carcinoma showed progression of disease or died, whereas no patients with NETs classified as benign or as having uncertain behavior showed local recurrence, disease progression, or died.

Declaration of interest: There is no conflict of interest that could be perceived as prejudicing the impartiality of the research reported.

Funding: This research did not receive any specific grant from any funding agency in the public, commercial, or not-for-profit sector.

Author contributions: This manuscript is the second part of M. B. Niederle's doctoral thesis 'Neuroendocrine tumors of the digestive tract in Austria' (N090 Endocrinology and Metabolism), for obtaining the academic title Doctor of Medical Science at the Medical University of Vienna.

Acknowledgements: The authors wish to thank Bettina Haidbauer for running the study secretariat and the members of the Austrian Society of Internal Medicine and Surgery for supporting this national study.

5.4.6 Tables

		WHO 2000	WHO 2010		
			NET G1	NET G2	NEC G3
WDET (1)	Benign (1a)	33/77 (42.9)	30/33 (90.9)	3/33 (9.1)	
	Uncertain (1b)	13/77 (16.9)	7/13 (53.8)	6/13 (46.2)	
		46/77 (59.7)^			
WDEC (2)		24/77 (31.2)	9/24 (37.5)	15/24 (62.5)	
PDEC (3)		7/77 (9.1)			7/7 (100)
			46/77 (59.1)	24/77 (31.2)	7/77 (9.1)

WDET: Well differentiated neuroendocrine tumor
WDEC: well differentiated endocrine carcinoma
PDEC: Poorly differentiated endocrine carcinoma
NET: neuroendocrine tumor

^ Data presented as n (%)

G1: mitotic count <2 per 10 high power fields (HPF) and/or ≤2% Ki67
G2: mitotic count 2-20 per 10 HPF and/or 3-20%Ki67 index
G3: mitotic count >20 per 10 HPF and/or 20% Ki67 index

Table 32 - Comparison of WHO 2000 [63] and WHO 2010 [69] using the example of 77 (27.8%) of 277 NETs documented within this clinical investigation

NET diagnosis in department of	Stomach	Duodenum/ ampulla	Pancreas	Prox./distal jejunum/Ileum	Appendix	Colon	Rectum	Total (%)
	65	16	33	44	59	20	40	277
Internal medicine	45 (69.2)^	10 (62.5)	6 (18.2)	6 (13.6)	1 (1.7)	8 (40.0)	14 (35.0)	90 (32.5)
Visceral surgery	20 (30.8)	6 (37.5)	22 (66.7)	36 (81.8)	50 (84.7)	12 (60.0)	16 (65.0)	180 (64.9)
Pediatric surgery					3 (5.1)			
Gynecology					4 (6.8)			
Urology					1 (1.7)			
Pathology			5 (15.2)	2 (4.5)				7 (2.5)
NET diagnosis by								
Endoscopy	63 (96.9)	13 (81.2)	2 (6.1)	9 (20.5)	1 (1.7)	11 (55.0)	36 (90.0)	135 (48.1)
Surgery	2 (3.1)	3 (18.8)	17 (51.5)	28 (63.6)	58 (98.3)	9 (45.0)	4 (10.0)	121 (43.7)
FNA (metastasis)			2 (6.1)	2 (4.5)				4 (1.4)
Autopsy			7 (21.2)	3 (6.8)				10 (3.6)
Pathology			5 (15.2)	2 (4.5)				7 (2.5)
Incidental diagnosis								
Information available	17/65 (26.2)	5/16 (31.3)	20/33 (60.6)	28/44 (36.4)	56/59 (94.9)	16/20 (80.0)	13/40 (32.5)	155/277 (56.0)
Incidentally diagnosed	3/17	1/5	0	6/28	55/56~	2/16	2/13	69/155 (44.5)
WHO 1a	3*	1**			35	1****	1+	41
WHO 1b					16		1++	17
WHO 2				6***	3#	1*****		7
WHO 3					1#			4

^ Data presented as n (%) , WHO World Health Organization classification.2000

Stomach *adenocarcinoma: n = 3; duodenum ** benign peptic ulcer: n = 1; **small intestine** ***acute bowel obstruction: n = 3; intestinal bleeding: n = 2; sigma resection (diverticulitis): n = 1; **appendix** ~ appendicitis (n = 36), during hemicolectomy (n = 4; indication for right hemicolectomy: adenoma ileocecal valve n =1; adenocarcinoma colon acendens: n = 1; pseudomembranous colitis/ischemia of cecal region: n = 1; adenocarcinoma cecum: n = 1), gynecological surgery (n = 4; ovarian cancer: n = 1; indication unknown n = 3); surgery because of ileus (n = 3; perforation of sigma diverticulitis: n = 1; reason unknown n = 2), rectum resection (n = 2; indication?), cholecystectomy (n = 1); surgery for Meckel diverticulum (n = 1; rupture of Meckel diverticulum with ileocecal resection), vascular aortic surgery (n = 1), or urological surgery (n = 1; cancer of the urinary bladder - radical cystectomy); # Goblet cell carcinoid: n = 4; **colon** ****adenocarcinoma in the colon: n = 1 *****acute colon obstruction (NET): n = 1;

Table 33 - Diagnosing department, diagnostic procedures, and incidental diagnosis of neuroendocrine tumors

Treatment	Stomach	Duodenum/ ampulla	Pancreas	Prox./distal jejunum/ileum	Appendix	Colon	Rectum	Total
Cases (n)	65	16	33	44	59	20	40	277
No information	20	5	3	12	3	4	11	58/277 (20.9)
Information available	45/65 (69.2)^	11/16 (68.8)	30/33 (90.9)	32/44 (72.3)	56/59 (94.9)	16/20 (80.0)	29/40 (72.5)	219/277 (79.1)
Surgery	15/45 (33.3)	5/11 (45.5)	20/30 (66.7)	28*/32 (87.5)	56/56 (100)	11/16 (68.8)	13/29 (44.8)	148*/219 (67.6)
Endoscopy	20/45 (44.4)	4/11 (36.4)	0	0	0	4/16 (25.0)	13/29 (44.8)	41/219 (18.7)
No intervention	10/45 (22.2)	2/11 (18.2)	10/30 (33.3)	4/32 (12.5)	0	1/16 (6.3)	3/29 (10.3)	30/219 (13.7)
WHO 1a	7	1	1				1	10
WHO 1b	1							1
WHO 2	2 (M pos 2)	1 (M pos 1)	6 (M pos 4)	4 (2**)(M pos 4)		1 (M pos 1)	2 (M pos 2)	14 (M pos 12)
WHO 3			3 (M pos 3)					5 (M pos 5)

^ data presented as n (%); *WHO* World Health Organization classification 2000
* cholecystectomy: primary NET in the ileum not removed;
** autopsy diagnosis.

Table 34 - Treatment modalities in patients with neuroendocrine tumors: surgery, endoscopy, no intervention

| Location | Details available/ total patients (%) | Surgical/endoscopic Intervention | n (%) | WHO classification |||||
| | | | | Well-differentiated ||| Poorly differentiated |
				WHO 1a benign 129/277	WHO 1b uncertain 44/277	WHO 2 malignant 86/277	WHO 3 malignant 18/277
	188/277 (67.9)						
Stomach	35/65 (53.8)	Polypectomy	9 (25.7)	8	1	-	-
		Mucosectomy	11 (31.3)	8	2	1	-
		Subtotal gastrectomy	5 (14.3)	2 (1+1*)	-	1	2
		Gastrectomy	10 (28.6)	4 (2+2**)	1	5	-
Duodenum	9/16 (56.3)	Polypectomy	4 (44.4)	2	2	-	-
		Local excision	2 (22.2)	1	1	-	-
		Subtotal gastrectomy	2 (22.2)	1~	-	1	-
		Whipple procedure	1 (11.1)	-	-	1	-
Pancreas	20/33 (60.6)	Enucleation	5 (25.0)	2	3	-	-
		Whipple procedure	5 (25.0)	-	1	4	-
		Left resection	7 (35.0)	-	-	7	-
		Central resection	1 (5.0)	-	1	-	-
		Gastroenterostomy	1 (5.0)	-	-	1	-
		Debulking	1 (5.0)	-	-	-	1
Small intestine	27/44 (61.4)	Segmental resection	13 (48.1)	1	-	12	-
		Ileocecal resection	7 (25.9)	1	-	6	-
		Right hemicolectomy	7 (25.9)	-	-	7	-
Appendix	56/59 (94.9)	Appendectomy	50 (89.3)	32	15	3+++	-
		Ileocecal resection	1 (1.8)	-	1++++	-	-
		Hemicolectomy	5 (8.9)	3+	-	2++	-
Re-operations	9/56 (16.1)	Appendectomy	1	-	-	1oo	-
		Ileocecal resection	7	-	1ooo	-	-
		Hemicolectomy	1	-	5	-	-
Colon	15/20 (75.0)	Polypectomy	4 (26.7)	4	-	3o	1o
		Hemicolectomy	9 (60.0)	1□	-	7	-
		Subtotal colectomy	1 (6.7)	1□	-	-	1□□
		Sigma resection	1 (6.7)	-	2	-	-
Rectum	26/40 (65.0)	Polypectomy	13 (50.0)	11	3	-	-
		Mucosectomy	8 (30.8)	5	-	-	-
		Rectal resection	5 (19.2)	2†	-	1	1

^ data presented as n (%)
Stomach *indication for subtotal gastrectomy – adenocarcinoma: n = 1; **indication for gastrectomy – adenocarcinoma: n = 2; **duodenum** ~indication for subtotal gastrectomy – peptic gastric ulcer; appendix Initial operations: + hemicolectomy: n = 3, ENETS T1N0M0: n = 3 (indication for right hemicolectomy – adenoma ileocecal valve n = 1; adenocarcinoma colon acendens: n = 1; pseudomembranous colitis/ischemia of cecal region: n = 1); ++hemicolectomy n = 2 (preoperative diagnosis by colonoscopy: n = 1; adenocarcinoma cecum: n = 1); +++ appendectomy: n = 1 T3N0M0 (tumor diameter 25 mm); ++++ileocecal resection: n = 1 (indication: perforated Meckel diverticulum); Reoperations (n = 9) ohemicolectomy: n = 7 (indication WHO/ENETS: WHO 1b/ pT3N0M0: n = 3; goblet cell carcinoid: n = 4 WHO 2/pT2N0M0: n = 2; WHO 2/pT3NXMX: n = 1; WHO 3/pT4N1M1: n = 1); oo local lymphadenectomy (following initial appendectomy in a pediatric patient): n = 1 (initial and re-operation: WHO 1b/pT3N0M0 25 mm; unclear margins); ooo ileocecal resection: n = 1 (WHO 1b/pT3N0M0; unclear resection margins after appendectomy T3N0M0: n = 1); **colon** □ WHO 1a/T1N0M0; □□ WHO 3 (30 mm) and synchronous colon cancer: n = 1; **rectum** WHO † 1a/T1N0M0: n = 2.

Table 35 - Endoscopic and surgical interventions in 188 patients in relation to WHO 2000 classification and NET location

Metastasis	Stomach	Duodenum/ ampulla	Pancreas	Prox./distal jejunum/ Jejunum/	Appendix	Colon	Rectum	Total
Patients with metastasis	8/11 (72.7)^	2/3 (66.7)	15/22 (68.2)	27/31 (87.1)	2/5 (40.0)	8/10 (80.0)	3/5 (60.0)	65/87 (74.7)
Lymph nodes	5	1	9	21	2	7	1	45/87 (51.7)
Liver	5	1	11	13		3	2	35 (40.2)
solitary	1	0	0	1	0	1	0	3
multiple	4	1	11	12	0	2	2	32
Peritoneum	2		1	6	1	1		11 (12.6)
Bone		1	2	1		1	1	4 (4.6)
Lung			2					2 (2.3)
Ovary			1					2 (2.3)
Brain			1					1 (1.1)
Both lymph nodes + distant metastasis	4	1	7	11	2	3		29 (33.3)

^ data presented as n (%)

Table 36 - Location of metastasis: 104/277 (37.5%) tumors classified as malignant (WHO 2 and 3) using the WHO criteria

NET location	Stomach	Duodenum/ampulla	Pancreas	Prox./distal jejunum/ileum	Appendix	Colon	Rectum	Total
Total	65	16	33	44	59	20	40	277
^	8/42 (19.0)	1/10 (10.0)	2/22 (8.9)	6/32 (18.0)	8/43 (18.6)	3/12 (23.1)	6/25 (24.0)	34/176 (19.3)
Additional malignancy								
Synchronous	6	0	1	0	6	2	6	21/41 (51.2)
Before	3	0	1	5	3	0	2	14/41 (34.1)
After	1	1	0	2	1	1	0	6 (14.6)
Total	10	1	2	7	10	3	8	41
Type of malignancy								
Adeno (GI)	6			1	4	2	6	19
Stomach	6						1	7
Colon/rectum				1	4	2	5	12
Adeno (NGI)	2		1	1	3	1	2	7
Breast	2			2	1			6
GIST								2
Lymphoma				2				2
Brain			1	1				2
Liver								1
Thyroid					1			1
Skin		1						1
NET					1			1

^ number of patients with information available / number of patients (%)
Adeno (GI): Adenocarcinoma (gastrointestinal); Adeno (NGI): Adenocarcinoma (non-gastrointestinal); GIST: Gastrointestinal stroma tumor

Table 37 - Additional malignancy: clinical data available in 176/277 (61.7%) patients with neuroendocrine tumors

	Stomach	Duodenum/ ampulla	Pancreas	Prox./distal jejunum/ ileum	Appendix	Colon	Rectum	Total
Cases	65	16	33	44	59	20	40	277
Malignant*	13/65 (20.0)	3/16 (18.8)	25/33 (75.8)	38/44 (86.4)	6/59 (10.2)	14/20 (70.0)	5/40 (12.5)	104/277 (37.5)
information available /malignant	10/13 (76.9)	2/3 (66.6)	18/25 (72.0)	25/38 (65.8)	5/6 (83.3)	7/14 (50.0)	3/5 (60.0)	70/104 (67.3)
No therapy	5/10 (50.0)	0/2	11/18 (61.1)	15/25 (60.0)	5/5 (100.0)	4/7 (57.1)	0/3	40/70 (57.1)
Somatostatin analogues	2/4	2/2	4/7	10/10	-	1/2	1/3	20/28 (70.8)
Interferon	1/3	0/2	1/4	4/10	-	1/2	0/3	7/24 (29.1)
Chemotherapy	1/4	0/2	3/3	1/8	-	2/3	3/3	10/23 (33.3)

^ data presented as n (%)
* World Health Organization classification 2000

Table 38 - Medical treatment of patients with neuroendocrine tumors

6. Conclusions

- Correct pathohistological diagnosis is the key to adequate treatment [103]. NETs occasionally simulate other endocrine tumours and lymphomas and therefore only tumours classified as NET by positive immunohistochemical staining for chromogranin A and/or synaptophysin were included in this prospective study; this is crucial for the correct diagnosis of this tumour entity.
- Using these strict criteria, the incidence of gastrointestinal NETs in a middle European country has been demonstrated for the first time, subdividing them into groups as recommended by the WHO. Standard cancer registries cannot reflect the true incidence, because benign tumours are omitted from many national registries [115].
- The presumptions by Klöppel [102, 120] that NETs are most frequently located in the stomach have been confirmed for the first time. NETs located in the stomach were followed by sites in the appendix, small intestine, rectum, pancreas and colon.
- According to the WHO 2000 classification [63], 46% of NETs were classified as benign, 43% as showing uncertain biological behaviour and 39% as showing malignant behaviour.
- Although some NETs show benign behaviour, all are potentially malignant. Using the recently proposed ENETS TNM classification [70, 71], a minority of gastrointestinal NETs were classified as Stage IIIB (N positive 11.0%; regional disease) and IV (N and/or M positive 23.8%; distant disease) at the time of diagnosis; this indicates a potentially incurable disease state.
- According to the proposed ENETS grading [70, 71] and the WHO classification 2010 [69], the majority of NETs were G1 (NET G1; 59.7%) and G2 (NET G2, 31.2%) independent of their staging. G3 tumours (Neuronedocrine Carcinoma) are very rare (9.1%).
- Because of their rarity and the often uncharacteristic clinical symptoms, clinicians include NETs very late in the differential diagnosis. Correct diagnosis and appropriate treatment are frequently difficult, even in expert settings.
- Endoscopic techniques are of highest relevance for diagnosis in the upper (stomach, duodenum) and lower (rectum, colon) gastrointestinal tract

- The majority of malignant tumors have already metastasized at time of diagnosis, mainly to lymph nodes.
- The majority of the pancreatic NETs may be non-functioning – this is either functioning tumours are not diagnosed as such (because of low appliance of specific serum testing for elevated hormonal levels) or former reports over-diagnose functioning pancreatic NETs due to center effects
- Endoscopic resection is an adequate therapeutic tool where applicable for small benign tumours especially in the stomach, duodenum, colon and rectum
- Radical surgical approach incl. lymph node resection is the key to treatment of malignant GEP-NETs

7. References

1. Medvei, V.C., *The History of Clinical Endocrinology.* 1993, The Parthenon Publishing Group. Carnforth: 551 pages.
2. Medvei, V.C., *Historical Introduction*, in *Clinical Endocrine Oncology;* Sheaves, R., Jenkins, P. and Wass, J.A.H. (eds). 1997, Blackwell Science. Oxford: p. 1-7,
3. Raju, T.N., *A mysterious something: the discovery of insulin and the 1923 Nobel Prize for Frederick G. Banting (1891-1941) and John J.R. Macleod (1876-1935).* Acta Paediatr, 2006. **95**(10): 1155-6.
4. Champaneria, M.C., et al., *Friedrich Feyrter: a precise intellect in a diffuse system.* Neuroendocrinology, 2006. **83**(5-6): 394-404.
5. Modlin, I.M., et al., *Evolution of the diffuse neuroendocrine system--clear cells and cloudy origins.* Neuroendocrinology, 2006. **84**(2): 69-82.
6. Modlin, I.M., et al., *Siegfried oberndorfer and the evolution of carcinoid disease.* Arch Surg, 2007. **142**(2): 187-97.
7. Oberndorfer, S., *Karzinoide Tumoren des Dünndarms.* Frankf Z Pathol, 1907. **1**: 426-432.
8. Masson, P., *La glande endocrine de l'intestin chez l'homme.* CR Acad Sci, 1914. **158**: 59-61.
9. Masson, P., *Carcinoids (argentaffin-cell tumors) and nerve hyperplasia of the appendicular mucosa.* Am J Path, 1928. **4**: 181-212.
10. Feyrter, F., *Über diffuse endocrine epitheliale Organe.* 1938, Barth. Leipzig: pages.
11. Zollinger, R.M.E.E.H., *Primary peptic ulcerations of the jejunum associated with islet cell tumors of the pancreas.* Ann Surg, 1955. **142**(4): 709–723.
12. Pearse, A.G., *The cytochemistry and ultrastructure of polypetide hormone-producing cells of the APUD series and the embryologic, physiologic and pathologic implications of the concept.* J Histochem Cytochem, 1969. **17**: 303-313.
13. Erdheim, J., *Zur normalen und pathologischen Histologie der Glandula thyreoidea, parathyroidea und Hypophysis.* Beit Z Path Anat Z Allg Path., 1903. **33**: 158-236.
14. Underdahl, L.O., Woolner, L.B., and Black, B.M., *Multiple endocrine adenomas: report of 8 cases in which the parathyroids, pituitary and pancreatic islets were involved.* J Clin Endocrin Metab, 1953. **13**: 20-47.
15. Wermer, P., *Genetic aspect of adenomatosis of endocrine glands.* Am J Med, 1954. **16**: 363-371.
16. Sipple, J.H., *The association of pheochromocytoma with carcinoma of the thyroid gland.* Am J Med, 1961. **31**: 163-66.
17. Williams, E.D. and Pollock, D.J., *Multiple mucosal neuromata with endocrine tumors: a syndrome allied to von Recklinghausen's disease.* J Pathol Bact, 1966. **91**: 71-80.
18. Steiner, A.L., Goodman, A.D., and Powers, S.R., *Study of a kindred with pheochromocytoma, medullary thyroid carcinoma, hyperparathyroidism, and Cushing's disease: multiple endocrine neoplasia, type 2.* Medicine (Baltimore), 1968. **47**: 371-409.
19. Carney, J.A., *Familial multiple endocrine neoplasia: the first 100 years.* Am J Surg Pathol, 2005. **29**(2): 254-74.

20. Andrew, A., Kramer, B., and Rawdon, B.B., *The origin of gut and pancreatic neuroendocrine (APUD) cells--the last word?* J Pathol, 1998. **186**(2): 117-8.
21. Wright, N.A., *The Origin of Gut Neuroendocrine Cells*, in *A Century of Advances in Neuroendocrine Tumor Biology and Treatment;* Modlin, I.M. and Öberg, K.(eds). 2007, Felsenstein C.C.C.P. Hannover: p. 156-63,
22. Altmann, H.W., *Die parafolliculäre Zelle der Schilddrüse und ihre Beziehungen zu der Gelben Zelle des Darmes.* Beitr Path Anat, 1940. **104**: 419-428.
23. Scothorne, R.J., *The borderland of embryology and pathology in the gut epithelium.* Histopathology, 1988. **13**(3): 355-9.
24. Winton, D.J. and Ponder, B.A., *Stem-cell organization in mouse small intestine.* Proc Biol Sci, 1990. **241**(1300): 13-8.
25. Thompson, M., et al., *Gastric endocrine cells share a clonal origin with other gut cell lineages.* Development, 1990. **110**(2): 477-81.
26. Novelli, M.R., et al., *Polyclonal origin of colonic adenomas in an XO/XY patient with FAP.* Science, 1996. **272**(5265): 1187-90.
27. Novelli, M., et al., *X-inactivation patch size in human female tissue confounds the assessment of tumor clonality.* Proc Natl Acad Sci U S A, 2003. **100**(6): 3311-4.
28. McDonald, S.A., et al., *Clonal expansion in the human gut: mitochondrial DNA mutations show us the way.* Cell Cycle, 2006. **5**(8): 808-11.
29. Leach, S.D., *Essential Elements of Enteroendocrine Evolution*, in *A Century of Advances in Neuroendocrine Tumor Biology and Treatment;* (eds). 2007, Felsenstein C.C.C.P. Hannover: p. 148-55,
30. Mellitzer, G., Jenny, M., and Gradwohl, G., *Neuroendocrine Cell Biology - Learning of Lineage*, in *A Century of Advances in Neuroendocrine Tumor Biology and Treatment;* Modlin, I.M. and Öberg, K. (eds). 2007, Felsenstein C.C.C.P. Hannover: p. 164-71,
31. Skipper, M. and Lewis, J., *Getting to the guts of enteroendocrine differentiation.* Nat Genet, 2000. **24**(1): 3-4.
32. Hocker, M. and Wiedenmann, B., *Molecular mechanisms of enteroendocrine differentiation.* Ann N Y Acad Sci, 1998. **859**: 160-74.
33. Drucker, D.J., *Gastrointestinal hormones and gut endocrine tumors*, in *Williams Textbook of Endocrinology;* Kronenberg, H.M., Melmed, S., Polonsky, K.S. and Larsen, P.R. (eds). 2008, Saunders Elsevier. Philadelphia: p. 1675-94,
34. Rindi, G., et al., *The "normal" endocrine cell of the gut: changing concepts and new evidences.* Ann N Y Acad Sci, 2004. **1014**: 1-12.
35. Wiedenmann, B., et al., *Molecular and cell biological aspects of neuroendocrine tumors of the gastroenteropancreatic system.* J Mol Med, 1998. **76**(9): 637-47.
36. Taupenot, L., Harper, K.L., and O'Connor, D.T., *The chromogranin-secretogranin family.* N Engl J Med, 2003. **348**(12): 1134-49.
37. Jahn, R., *Principles of exocytosis and membrane fusion.* Ann N Y Acad Sci, 2004. **1014**: 170-8.
38. Silbernagl, S. and Despopoulos, A., *Taschenatlas der Physiologie.* 2003, Thieme. Stuttgart: 436 pages.
39. Gustafsson, B., et al., *The Enterochromaffin Cell*, in *A Century of Advances in Neuroendocrine Tumor Biology and Treatment;* Modlin, I.M. and Öberg, K. (eds). 2007, Felsenstein C.C.C.P. Hannover: p. 178-91,

40. Sternini, C., Anselmi, L., and Rozengurt, E., *Enteroendocrine cells: a site of 'taste' in gastrointestinal chemosensing.* Curr Opin Endocrinol Diabetes Obes, 2008. **15**(1): 73-8.
41. Wilding, J.P.H., Ghatei, M.A., and Bloom, S.R., *Hormones of the Gastrointestinal Tract*, in *Endocrinology, Volume 3; DeGroot, L. et al*(eds). 1995, W.B. Saunders. Philadelphia: p. 2870-93,
42. Cegla, J., Tan, T.M., and Bloom, S.R., *Gut-brain cross-talk in appetite regulation.* Curr Opin Clin Nutr Metab Care, 2010. **13**(5): 588-93.
43. Khan, W.I. and Ghia, J.E., *Gut hormones: emerging role in immune activation and inflammation.* Clin Exp Immunol, 2010. **161**(1): 19-27.
44. Buse, J.B., Polonsky, K.S., and Buran, C.F., *Type 2 Diabetes Mellitus*, in *Williams Textbook of Endocrinology;* Kronenberg, H.M., Melmed, S., Polonsky, K.S. and Larsen, P.R. (eds). 2008, Saunders Elsevier. Philadelphia: p. 1329-90,
45. Green, G.M. and Reeve, J.R., Jr., *Unique activities of cholecystokinin-58; physiological and pathological relevance.* Curr Opin Endocrinol Diabetes Obes, 2008. **15**(1): 48-53.
46. Edholm, T., et al., *Differential incretin effects of GIP and GLP-1 on gastric emptying, appetite, and insulin-glucose homeostasis.* Neurogastroenterol Motil, 2010. **22**(11): 1191-200, e315.
47. Drucker, D.J., *Gut adaptation and the glucagon-like peptides.* Gut, 2002. **50**(3): 428-35.
48. Wynne, K., et al., *Subcutaneous oxyntomodulin reduces body weight in overweight and obese subjects: a double-blind, randomized, controlled trial.* Diabetes, 2005. **54**(8): 2390-5.
49. Poitras, P. and Peeters, T.L., *Motilin.* Curr Opin Endocrinol Diabetes Obes, 2008. **15**(1): 54-7.
50. Bousquet, C., et al., *Somatostatin Receptors: Current and Future Concepts*, in *A Century of Advances in Neuroendocrine Tumor Biology and Treatment;* Modlin, I.M. and Öberg, K. (eds). 2007, Felsenstein C.C.C.P. Hannover: p. 232-240,
51. Chandarana, K. and Batterham, R., *Peptide YY.* Curr Opin Endocrinol Diabetes Obes, 2008. **15**(1): 65-72.
52. Gonzalez, N., et al., *Bombesin-related peptides and their receptors: recent advances in their role in physiology and disease states.* Curr Opin Endocrinol Diabetes Obes, 2008. **15**(1): 58-64.
53. Duerr, E.-M. and Chung, D.C., *Molecular Genetics of Pancreatic Neuroendocrine Tumors*, in *A Century of Advances in Neuroendocrine Tumor Biology and Treatment;* Modlin, I.M. and Öberg, K.(eds). 2007, Felsenstein C.C.C.P. Hannover: p. 210-7,
54. Perren, A., Anlauf, M., and Komminoth, P., *Molecular profiles of gastroenteropancreatic endocrine tumors.* Virchows Arch, 2007. **451 Suppl 1**: S39-46.
55. Capurso, G., et al., *Gene expression profiles of progressive pancreatic endocrine tumours and their liver metastases reveal potential novel markers and therapeutic targets.* Endocr Relat Cancer, 2006. **13**(2): 541-58.
56. Terris, B., et al., *Comparative genomic hybridization analysis of sporadic neuroendocrine tumors of the digestive system.* Genes Chromosomes Cancer, 1998. **22**(1): 50-6.

57. Lollgen, R.M., et al., *Chromosome 18 deletions are common events in classical midgut carcinoid tumors.* Int J Cancer, 2001. **92**(6): 812-5.
58. Cotran, R.S., et al., *Robbins Pathologic Basis of Disease, 5th edition.* 1994, W.B. Saunders Company. Philadelphia: pages.
59. Barakat, M.T., Meeran, K., and Bloom, S.R., *Neuroendocrine tumours.* Endocr Relat Cancer, 2004. **11**(1): 1-18.
60. Kloppel, G., *Neuroendokrine Tumoren des Gastrointestinaltrakts.* Pathologe, 2003. **24**(4): 287-96.
61. Gustafsson, B.I., Kidd, M., and Modlin, I.M., *Neuroendocrine tumors of the diffuse neuroendocrine system.* Curr Opin Oncol, 2008. **20**(1): 1-12.
62. Kloppel, G., Perren, A., and Heitz, P.U., *The gastroenteropancreatic neuroendocrine cell system and its tumors: the WHO classification.* Ann N Y Acad Sci, 2004. **1014**: 13-27.
63. Solcia, E., Kloppel, G., and Sobin, L. eds, *Histological Typing of Endocrine Tumours.* 2nd Edition. World Health Organization International Histological Classification of Tumours. 2000, Springer. Berlin: 156
64. Plockinger, U., et al., *Guidelines for the diagnosis and treatment of neuroendocrine gastrointestinal tumours. A consensus statement on behalf of the European Neuroendocrine Tumour Society (ENETS).* Neuroendocrinology, 2004. **80**(6): 394-424.
65. Reubi, J.C., *Peptide receptor expression in GEP-NET.* Virchows Arch, 2007. **451 Suppl 1**: S47-50.
66. Williams, E.D. and Sandler, M., *The classification of carcinoid tumours.* Lancet, 1963. **1**(7275): 238-9.
67. Schmitt-Gräff, A., Nitschke, R., and Wiedenmann, B., *Gastroenteropankreatische neuroendokrine/endokrine Tumoren - Aktuelle pathologisch-diagnostische Sicht.* Pathologe, 2001. **22**: 105-13.
68. Vilar, E., et al., *Chemotherapy and role of the proliferation marker Ki-67 in digestive neuroendocrine tumors.* Endocr Relat Cancer, 2007. **14**(2): 221-32.
69. Bosman, F., et al. eds, *WHO Classification of Tumours of the Digestive System.* 2010, IARC Press. Lyon: 418
70. Rindi, G., et al., *TNM staging of foregut (neuro)endocrine tumors: a consensus proposal including a grading system.* Virchows Arch, 2006. **449**(4): 395-401.
71. Rindi, G., et al., *TNM staging of midgut and hindgut (neuro) endocrine tumors: a consensus proposal including a grading system.* Virchows Arch, 2007. **451**(4): 757-62.
72. Sobin, L., Gospodarowicz, M., and Wittekind, C. eds, *UICC: TNM classification of malignant tumours, 7th edition.* 2009, Wiley-Blackwell. Oxford
73. Kloppel, G., et al., *The ENETS and AJCC/UICC TNM classifications of the neuroendocrine tumors of the gastrointestinal tract and the pancreas: a statement.* Virchows Arch, 2010. **456**(6): 595-7.
74. Pape, U.F., et al., *Prognostic relevance of a novel TNM classification system for upper gastroenteropancreatic neuroendocrine tumors.* Cancer, 2008. **113**(2): 256-65.
75. Scarpa, A., et al., *Pancreatic endocrine tumors: improved TNM staging and histopathological grading permit a clinically efficient prognostic stratification of patients.* Mod Pathol, 2010. **23**(6): 824-33.
76. Volante, M., et al., *Goblet cell carcinoids and other mixed neuroendocrine/nonneuroendocrine neoplasms.* Virchows Arch, 2007. **451 Suppl 1**: S61-9.

77. Kloppel, G., et al., *Site-specific biology and pathology of gastroenteropancreatic neuroendocrine tumors.* Virchows Arch, 2007. **451 Suppl 1**: S9-27.
78. Ruszniewski, P., et al., *Well-differentiated gastric tumors/carcinomas.* Neuroendocrinology, 2006. **84**(3): 158-64.
79. Nilsson, O., et al., *Poorly differentiated carcinomas of the foregut (gastric, duodenal and pancreatic).* Neuroendocrinology, 2006. **84**(3): 212-5.
80. Jensen, R.T., et al., *Well-differentiated duodenal tumor/carcinoma (excluding gastrinomas).* Neuroendocrinology, 2006. **84**(3): 165-72.
81. Jensen, R.T., et al., *Gastrinoma (duodenal and pancreatic).* Neuroendocrinology, 2006. **84**(3): 173-82.
82. Falconi, M., et al., *Well-differentiated pancreatic nonfunctioning tumors/carcinoma.* Neuroendocrinology, 2006. **84**(3): 196-211.
83. de Herder, W.W., et al., *Well-differentiated pancreatic tumor/carcinoma: insulinoma.* Neuroendocrinology, 2006. **84**(3): 183-8.
84. O'Toole, D., et al., *Rare functioning pancreatic endocrine tumors.* Neuroendocrinology, 2006. **84**(3): 189-95.
85. Schmitt, A.M., et al., *WHO 2004 criteria and CK19 are reliable prognostic markers in pancreatic endocrine tumors.* Am J Surg Pathol, 2007. **31**(11): 1677-82.
86. Plöckinger, U., *Neuroendokrine gastrointestinale Tumoren.* 2007, Uni-Med Verlag. Bremen: 125 pages.
87. Kloppel, G. and Anlauf, M., *Pancreatic Endocrine Tumors.* Pathology Case Reviews, 2006. **11**(6): 256-67.
88. Eriksson, B., et al., *Consensus guidelines for the management of patients with digestive neuroendocrine tumors--well-differentiated jejunal-ileal tumor/carcinoma.* Neuroendocrinology, 2008. **87**(1): 8-19.
89. Ahlman, H., et al., *Poorly-differentiated endocrine carcinomas of midgut and hindgut origin.* Neuroendocrinology, 2008. **87**(1): 40-6.
90. Plockinger, U., et al., *Consensus guidelines for the management of patients with digestive neuroendocrine tumours: well-differentiated tumour/carcinoma of the appendix and goblet cell carcinoma.* Neuroendocrinology, 2008. **87**(1): 20-30.
91. Ramage, J.K., et al., *Consensus guidelines for the management of patients with digestive neuroendocrine tumours: well-differentiated colon and rectum tumour/carcinoma.* Neuroendocrinology, 2008. **87**(1): 31-9.
92. Anlauf, M., et al., *Hereditary neuroendocrine tumors of the gastroenteropancreatic system.* Virchows Arch, 2007. **451 Suppl 1**: S29-38.
93. O'Toole, D., et al., *ENETS Consensus Guidelines for the Standards of Care in Neuroendocrine Tumors: biochemical markers.* Neuroendocrinology, 2009. **90**(2): 194-202.
94. Plockinger, U. and Wiedenmann, B., *Treatment of gastroenteropancreatic neuroendocrine tumors.* Virchows Arch, 2007. **451 Suppl 1**: S71-80.
95. Steinmuller, T., et al., *Consensus guidelines for the management of patients with liver metastases from digestive (neuro)endocrine tumors: foregut, midgut, hindgut, and unknown primary.* Neuroendocrinology, 2008. **87**(1): 47-62.
96. Berge, T. and Linell, F., *Carcinoid tumours. Frequency in a defined population during a 12-year period.* Acta Pathol Microbiol Scand [A], 1976. **84**(4): 322-30.
97. Godwin, J.D., 2nd, *Carcinoid tumors. An analysis of 2,837 cases.* Cancer, 1975. **36**(2): 560-9.

98. Modlin, I.M., Lye, K.D., and Kidd, M., *A 5-decade analysis of 13,715 carcinoid tumors.* Cancer, 2003. **97**(4): 934-59.
99. Hemminki, K. and Li, X., *Incidence trends and risk factors of carcinoid tumors: a nationwide epidemiologic study from Sweden.* Cancer, 2001. **92**(8): 2204-10.
100. Levi, F., et al., *Epidemiology of carcinoid neoplasms in Vaud, Switzerland, 1974-97.* Br J Cancer, 2000. **83**(7): 952-5.
101. Soga, J., *Carcinoids of the small intestine: a statistical evaluation of 1102 cases collected from the literature.* J Exp Clin Cancer Res, 1997. **16**(4): 353-63.
102. Kloppel, G., *Tumour biology and histopathology of neuroendocrine tumours.* Best Pract Res Clin Endocrinol Metab, 2007. **21**(1): 15-31.
103. Kloppel, G., et al., *ENETS Consensus Guidelines for the Standards of Care in Neuroendocrine Tumors: towards a standardized approach to the diagnosis of gastroenteropancreatic neuroendocrine tumors and their prognostic stratification.* Neuroendocrinology, 2009. **90**(2): 162-6.
104. Parkin, D.M., et al. eds, *Cancer Incidence in Five Continents Vol. VIII.* 2003, IARC Scientific Publications. Lyon: 781.155
105. Doll, R., Payne, P., and Waterhouse, J. eds, *Cancer Incidence in Five Continents: A Technical Report.* 1966, Springer-Verlag (for UICC) Berlin: 244
106. Segi, M., et al., *The age-adjusted death rates for malignant neoplasms in some selected sites in 23 countries in 1954-1955 and their geographical correlation.* Tohoku J Exp Med, 1960. **72**: 91-103.
107. Hauso, O., et al., *Neuroendocrine tumor epidemiology: contrasting Norway and North America.* Cancer, 2008. **113**(10): 2655-64.
108. Yao, J.C., et al., *One hundred years after "carcinoid": epidemiology of and prognostic factors for neuroendocrine tumors in 35,825 cases in the United States.* J Clin Oncol, 2008. **26**(18): 3063-72.
109. Klein, R.J. and Schoenborn, C.A., *Age adjustment using the 2000 projected U.S. population.* Healthy People 2000 Stat Notes, 2001(20): 1-9.
110. Kloppel, G., *Neuroendocrine tumors (2007): Oberndorfer's legacy.* Virchows Arch, 2007. **451 Suppl 1**: S1.
111. Taal, B.G. and Visser, O., *Epidemiology of neuroendocrine tumours.* Neuroendocrinology, 2004. **80 Suppl 1**: 3-7.
112. Berge, T. and Linell, F., *Carcinoid tumours. Frequency in a defined population during a 12-year period.* Acta Pathol Microbiol Scand, 1976. **84**(4): 322-30.
113. Helland, S.K., Prosch, A.M., and Viste, A., *Carcinoid tumours in the gastrointestinal tract--a population-based study from Western Norway.* Scand J Surg, 2006. **95**(3): 158-61.
114. Ito, T., et al., *Epidemiological study of gastroenteropancreatic neuroendocrine tumors in Japan.* J Gastroenterol, 2010. **45**(2): 234-243.
115. Gatta, G., et al., *Survival from rare cancer in adults: a population-based study.* Lancet Oncol, 2006. **7**(2): 132-40.
116. Klimstra, D.S., et al., *Pathology Reporting of Neuroendocrine Tumors: Application of the Delphic Consensus Process to the Development of a Minimum Pathology Data Set.* Am J Surg Pathol, 2010. **34**: 300-313.
117. Crocetti, E., Buiatti, E., and Amorosi, A., *Epidemiology of carcinoid tumours in central Italy.* Eur J Epidemiol, 1997. **13**(3): 357-9.
118. Newton, J.N., et al., *The epidemiology of carcinoid tumours in England and Scotland.* Br J Cancer, 1994. **70**(5): 939-42.

119. Maroun, J., et al., *Guidelines for the diagnosis and management of carcinoid tumours. Part 1: the gastrointestinal tract. A statement from a Canadian National Carcinoid Expert Group.* Curr Oncol, 2006. **13**(2): 67-76.
120. Kloppel, G. and Clemens, A., *The biological relevance of gastric neuroendocrine tumors.* Yale J Biol Med, 1996. **69**(1): 69-74.
121. Lombard-Bohas, C., et al., *Thirteen-month registration of patients with gastroenteropancreatic endocrine tumours in France.* Neuroendocrinology, 2009. **89**(2): 217-22.
122. Maggard, M.A., O'Connell, J.B., and Ko, C.Y., *Updated population-based review of carcinoid tumors.* Ann Surg, 2004. **240**(1): 117-22.
123. Li, A.F., et al., *A 35-year retrospective study of carcinoid tumors in Taiwan: differences in distribution with a high probability of associated second primary malignancies.* Cancer, 2008. **112**(2): 274-83.
124. Rindi, G., et al., *Gastric carcinoids and neuroendocrine carcinomas: pathogenesis, pathology, and behavior.* World J Surg, 1996. **20**(2): 168-72.
125. Halfdanarson, T.R., et al., *Pancreatic endocrine neoplasms: epidemiology and prognosis of pancreatic endocrine tumors.* Endocr Relat Cancer, 2008. **15**(2): 409-27.
126. Modlin, I.M. and Sandor, A., *An analysis of 8305 cases of carcinoid tumors.* Cancer, 1997. **79**(4): 813-29.
127. Niederle, M.B., et al., *Gastro-entero-pancreatic neuroendocrine tumours - the current incidence and staging based on the WHO and ENETS classification.* Endocr Relat Cancer, 2010. **17**: 909-18.
128. Schindl, M., et al., *Is the new classification of neuroendocrine pancreatic tumors of clinical help?* World J Surg, 2000. **24**(11): 1312-8.
129. Schindl, M., et al., *Treatment of small intestinal neuroendocrine tumors: is an extended multimodal approach justified?* World J Surg, 2002. **26**(8): 976-84.
130. Landerholm, K., Falkmer, S., and Jarhult, J., *Epidemiology of small bowel carcinoids in a defined population.* World J Surg, 2010. **34**(7): 1500-5.
131. Aggarwal, G., Obideen, K., and Wehbi, M., *Carcinoid tumors: what should increase our suspicion?* Cleve Clin J Med, 2008. **75**(12): 849-55.
132. Pape, U.F., et al., *Survival and clinical outcome of patients with neuroendocrine tumors of the gastroenteropancreatic tract in a german referral center.* Ann N Y Acad Sci, 2004. **1014**: 222-33.
133. Ploeckinger, U., et al., *The German NET-registry: an audit on the diagnosis and therapy of neuroendocrine tumors.* Neuroendocrinology, 2009. **90**(4): 349-63.
134. Marshall, J.B. and Bodnarchuk, G., *Carcinoid tumors of the gut. Our experience over three decades and review of the literature.* J Clin Gastroenterol, 1993. **16**(2): 123-9.
135. Pinchot, S.N., et al., *Carcinoid tumors.* Oncologist, 2008. **13**(12): 1255-69.
136. Rindi, G., et al., *Three subtypes of gastric argyrophil carcinoid and the gastric neuroendocrine carcinoma: a clinicopathologic study.* Gastroenterology, 1993. **104**(4): 994-1006.
137. Borch, K., et al., *Gastric carcinoids: biologic behavior and prognosis after differentiated treatment in relation to type.* Ann Surg, 2005. **242**(1): 64-73.
138. Schindl, M., Kaserer, K., and Niederle, B., *Treatment of gastric neuroendocrine tumors: the necessity of a type-adapted treatment.* Arch Surg, 2001. **136**(1): 49-54.

139. Deschamps, L. and Couvelard, A., *Endocrine tumors of the appendix: a pathologic review.* Arch Pathol Lab Med, 2010. **134**(6): 871-5.
140. Schindl, M., et al., *Stage-dependent therapy of rectal carcinoid tumors.* World J Surg, 1998. **22**(6): 628-33; discussion 634.
141. Fendrich, V., et al., *Multiple primary malignancies in patients with sporadic pancreatic endocrine tumors.* J Surg Oncol, 2008. **97**(7): 592-5.
142. Habal, N., Sims, C., and Bilchik, A.J., *Gastrointestinal carcinoid tumors and second primary malignancies.* J Surg Oncol, 2000. **75**(4): 310-6.
143. Tichansky, D.S., et al., *Risk of second cancers in patients with colorectal carcinoids.* Dis Colon Rectum, 2002. **45**(1): 91-7.
144. Brune, M., et al., *Neuroendocrine tumors of the gastrointestinal tract (NETGI) and second primary malignancies--which is dominant?* Dtsch Med Wochenschr, 2003. **128**(46): 2413-7.

8. Appendices

The author wish to thank Bettina Haidbauer for running the study secretariat, the members of the Austrian Society of Clinical Pathology and the members of the Austrian Society of Internal Medicine and Surgery for supporting this national study.

8.1 Appendix A: List of Austrian institutes of pathology and supporting pathologists

	Hospital	Chairman (during study period)	Pathologist	Reported Tumours (n)
1	Med Uni Vienna	D. Kerjaschki	K. Kaserer	21
2	Med Uni Innsbruck	G. Mikuz	Ch. Ensinger	22
3	Med Uni Graz*	H. Denk	C. Langner	43
4	Rudolfstiftung	H. Feichtinger	H. Feichtinger	0
5	SMZ-Süd (KFJ)	M. Klimpfinger	M. Klimpfinger	8
6	KH Hietzing	U. Walter	W. Ulrich	6
7	Hanusch KH	A. Nader	E. Herran	1
8	Baumgartner Höhe**	F. Lintner	F. Lintner	0
9	KES	N. Neuhold	N. Neuhold	1
10	Wilheminen Spital	K. Kofler	Ch. Dellinger	11
11	SMZ-Ost	Angelika Reiner	S. Grillenberger	11
12	KH Oberwart***	G. Böhm	G. Böhm	0
13	LKH Klagenfurt	H. Rogatsch	H. Rogatsch	18
14	LKH Villach	G. Alpi	G. Alpi	4
15	LKH Krems	W. Öhlinger	W. Öhlinger	3
16	KH St. Pölten	R. Sedivy	H. Bankl	3
17	KH Wr. Neustadt	W. Stiglbauer	W. Stiglbauer	6

18	KH Amstetten	F. Pantucek	F. Pantucek	3
19	Waldviertelklinikum Horn	O. Braun	O. Braun	3
20	KH Mistelbach	Ch. Freibauer	Ch. Freibauer	4
21	LKH Mödling	S. Naude	S. Naude	4
22	AKH Linz	G. Syre	G. Syre	8
23	KH Barmh. Schwestern Linz	W. Sega	P. Niedermoser	20
24	Landes-Nervenklinik Wagner-Jauregg Linz****	R. Silye	R. Silye	0
25	LKH Steyr	J. Feichtinger	A. Loidl	8
26	KH Barmh. Schwestern Wels	A. Haidenthaler	W. Höbling	22
27	KH Barmh. Schwestern Ried	G. Brinninger	G. Brinninger	1
28	LKH Vöcklabruck	H. Gogl	K. Fuchs	8
29	LKH Salzburg	O. S. Dietze	C. Hauser-	5
30	KH Schwarzach	A. Hittmair	A. Hittmair	2
31	LKH Feldkirch	F. Offner	F. Offner	10
32	LKH Leoben	G. Leitner	F. Tamos, F. Leitner	8
33	LKH Graz West	S. Lax	S. Lax	13
34	Rudolfinerhaus~	N. Neuhold	N. Neuhold	0
35	Patho.-Histolog. u. Zytolog.-Med.u. chem.Labordiagn. Prim. Dr. Braun~	O. Braun	O. Braun	0
36	Patholog.-histolog.-u. zytolog. Laboratorium - Leibl~	W. Leibl	W. Leibl	0
37	Labor Alsergrung (Birkmayer Labor & MEDINFO GmbH)~	J. Birkmayer	J. Birkmayer	0
38	Labor Kosak~	D. Kosak	D. Kosak	8
39	Med.-diagn. Laboratorium f. Zytologie und Histologie – Dr. Ulm	Ch. Wüstinger	Ch. Wüstinger	0
40	Labor Kerjaschki~	D. Kerjaschki	K. Kaserer	8
41	Beck Dr/Dr Haider GesmbH~	E. Beck	E. Beck	0

* 15 other hospitals are affiliated to this pathological institute
**Centre of Pulmonology
**** Centre of Neurosurgery
*** affiliated to 40
~ Private Institutes – two of eight institutes diagnosed GEP- NETs in the study period

8.2 Appendix B: List of participating clinical institutes and supporting physicians

Province	Hospital	Department	Chairman (2005/6)	Contact Person
Vienna	Wilhelminenspital	1. Chirurgische Abteilung	G. Hagmüller	G. Hagmüller
Vienna	Wilhelminenspital	2. Chirurgische Abteilung	K. Glaser	K. Schönau
Vienna	Wilhelminenspital	4. Medizinische Abteilung	M. Gschwantler	Gschwantler
Vienna	Med. Uni. Wien	Allgemeinchirurgie	R. Jakesz	
Vienna	Med. Uni. Wien	Abteillung für Innere Medizin IV/Gastroenterologie	A. Gangl	
Vienna	Rudolfsstiftung	4. Medizinische Abteilung	W. Weiss	. W. Weiss
Vienna	Kaiserin-Elisabeth-Spital	Chirurgische Abteilung	M. Hermann	M. Hermann
Vienna	Kaiser-Franz-Josef-Spital, SMZ Süd	Chirurgische Abteilung	J. Karner	T. Hoblaj
Vienna	Krankenhaus Hietzing	1. Medizinische Abteilung	H. Brunner	N. Zwerina
Vienna	Krankenhaus Göttlicher Heiland	Chirurgische Abteilung	V. Grablowitz	B. Obermaier
Vienna	Krankenhaus St. Elisabeth	Chirurgische Abteilung	M. Glöckler	M. Glöckler
Vienna	Krankenhaus Barmherzige Brüder	Chirurgische Abteilung	F. Herbst	F. Herst
Vienna	Krankenhaus Barmherzige Schwestern	Chirurgische Abteilung	M. Wunderlich	M. Lechner
Vienna	Ordination Primarius Dr. L. Cik, Wien		L. Cik	L. Cik
Vienna	SMZ Ost	2. Medizinische Abteilung	W. Hinterberger	R. Rucksner
Vienna	SMZ Ost	Chirurgische Abteilung	R. Schiessel	Dr. Hoffmann
Upper Austria	Klinikum Wels-Grieskirchen	Abteilung für Innere Medzin 1	P. Knoflach	P. Knoflach
Upper Austria	Klinikum Wels-Grieskirchen	2. Chirurgische Abteilung	T. Sautner	T. Sautner
Upper Austria	LKH Gmunden	Chirurgische Abteilung	R. Rieger	R. Rieger
Upper Austria	Krankenhaus Braunau	Innere Medizin 2	K. Täuber	K. Täuber
Lower Austria	LKH Mistelbauch	1. Medizinische Abteilung	O. Traindl	. O. Traindl
Lower Austria	LKH Wiener Neustadt	Chirurgische Abteilung	F. Längle	E. Bareck
Lower Austria	LKH Hollabrunn	Chirurgische Abteilung	K.Dittrich	K. Dittrich
Lower Austria	LKH Amstetten	Chirurgische Abteilung	F. Schmöller	F. Schmöller
Lower Austria	LKH St. Pölten	Chirurgische Abteilung	G. Salem	M. Sperlich
Lower Austria	LKH Mödling	Abteilung für Innere Medizin	F.X. Roithinger	F.X. Roithinger
Burgenland	Krankenhaus Kittsee	Chirurgische Abteilung	L. Bastian	L. Bastian
Styria	LKH Graz West	Chirurgische Abteilung	P. Steindorfer	. P. Steindorfer
Styria	LKH Judenburg-Knittelfeld	Medizinische Abteilung	W. Rainer	W. Rainer

Styria	LKH Leoben	Chirurgische Abteilung	H. Rabl	H. Rabl
Styria	LKH Leoben	Department für Gastroenterologie	K. Jilek	K. Jilek
Styria	LKH Mürzzuschlag	Chirurgische Abteilung	R. Schrittwieser	R. Schrittwieser
Styria	Ordination Dr. A. Pataki, Graz		A. Pataki	A. Pataki
Styria	Ordination Dr. H. Riegler, Rudersdorf		H. Riegler	H. Riegler
Styria	LKH Feldbach	Gynäkologische Abteilung	H. Hofmann	H. Hofmann
Styria	LKH Wagna	Medizinische Abteilung	H. Leskowschek	H. Leskowschek
Styria	LKH Weiz	Chirurgische Abteilung	K. Gruber	K. Gruber
Styria	Med. Uni. Graz	Medizinische Abteilung	G. Krejs	G. Krejs, Th. Hinterleitner
Corinthia	LKH Klagenfurt	Abteilung für Allgemein- und Viszeralchirurgie	Dr. M. Starlinger	M. Starlinger
Corinthia	LKH Klagenfurt	Innere Medizin 2	DDr. G. Grimm	A. Hebenstreit
Corinthia	Krankenhaus Waiern	Medizinische Abteilung	R. Gaugeler	R. Gaugeler
Corinthia	Krankenhaus Barmherzige Brüder St. Veit/Glan	Chirurgische Abteilung	J. Tschmelitsch	J. Tschmelitsch
Corinthia	Krankenhaus Barmherzige Brüder St. Veit/Glan	Abteilung für Innere Medizin	F. Siebert	M. Tomka
Corinthia	LKH Wolfsburg	Medizinische Abteilung	W. Fortunat	D. Plamenig
Corinthia	Ordination Dr. H. Fellinger, Klagenfurt		H. Fellinger	H. Fellinger
Corinthia	Ordination Dr. W. Weitensfelder		W. Weitensfelder	
Corinthia	Krankenhaus Elisabethinen Klagenfurt	Chirurgische Abteilung	G. Smolnig	G. Smolnig
Corinthia	Privatklinik Warmbad Villach	Chirurgische Abteilung	G. Zalaudek	G. Zalaudek
Tyrol	Krankenhaus Lienz	Abteilung für Innere Medizin	P. Lechleitner	L. Köck
Tyrol	Krankenhaus Lienz	Chirurgische Abteilung	M. Müller	M. Müller
Tyrol	Krankenhaus Kufstein	Chirurgische Abteilung	B. Spechtenhauser	J. Wiegele
Tyrol	Krankenhaus Kufstein	Abteilung für Innere Medizin	K. Gattringer	K. Gattringer
Tyrol	Krankenhaus Hall	Chirurgische Abteilung	D. E. Steiner	D. E. Steiner
Tyrol	Krankenhaus Zams	Chirurgische Abteilung	P. Sandbichler	P. Sandbichler
Tyrol	Krankenhaus Schwaz	Chirurgische Abteilung	G. Wetscher	G. Wetscher
Tyrol	Med. Uni. Innsbruck	Universitätsklinik für Viszeral-, Transplantations- und Thoraxchirurgie	R. Magreiter	R. Prommegger
Tyrol	Med. Uni. Innsbruck	Universitätsklinik für Innere Medizin 2	W. Vogel	W. Vogel
Vorarlberg	Ordination Dr. F. Reichsöllner		F. Reichsöllner	
Vorarlberg	LKH Bludenz	Chirurgische Abteilung	M. Scheyer	M. Scheyer
Vorarlberg	LKH Bludenz	Abteilung f. Innere Medizin	D. Striberski	D. Striberski
Vorarlberg	LKH Bregenz	Chirurgische Abteilung	D. Wohlgenannt	K. Zahel
Vorarlberg	LKH Feldkirch	Abteilung f. Innere Medizin	H. Drexel	Th. Flatz

Vorarlberg	LKH Feldkirch	Chirurgische Abteilung	E. Wenzl	E. Wenzl
Salzburg	LKH Salzburg	Chirurgische Abteilung	D. Öfner	P. Sungler

8.3 Appendix C: Pathological Report Form

GEP - NET – Inzidenz in Österreich

Anhang A: Teil 1

Pathologisches Institut:	
Institutseigene Histo-Protokoll Nr.	
Datum der Diagnose: TTMMJJJJ	
Patient: * zutreffendes bitte markieren	Männlich O Weiblich O Geb.-Dat.: TTMMJJJJ Initialen:(NN/VN) _____
Lokalisation* : * zutreffendes bitte markieren	Pankreas O Meckelsches Divertikel O Ösophagus O Appendix O Magen O Colon O Duodenum O Rektum O Jejunum O Leber O Ileum O
Präparat:	Operationspräparat O Biopsie O Autopsie O
WHO Klassifikation: * zutreffendes bitte markieren	Hoch differenzierter NE Tumor - gutartig O Hoch differenziertes NE Karzinom O Hoch differenzierter NE Tumor – unklare Dignität O Undifferenziertes (kleinzelliges) NE Karzinom O
Größe in mm:	_____ mm
Immunhistochemie: * zutreffendes bitte markieren	Chromogranin A O Synaptophysin O
Hormon Nachweis: optional	
Proliferationsindex: optional	
Zuweisende klinische Abteilung: (Kontaktperson)	
Bemerkungen:	

8.4 Appendix D: Clinical questionnaire

Studienkennzahl:	Erfassungsdatum:

A Stammdaten

A.1 Allgemeines

Name:(NN/VN):	Geschlecht: ☐ w ☐ m
Geburtsdatum:	
Patient/in verstorben: ☐ ja ☐ nein (weiter bei A.3)	

A.2 Sterbedaten

Sterbedatum:
Todesursache:

Todesursache gesichert: ☐ ja ☐ nein	Tumorassoziiert (neuroendokriner Tumor): ☐ ja ☐ nein

A.3 Hauptdiagnose

Zufallsbefund: ☐ Ja ☐ Nein	Diagnosedatum:
Pathologisches Institut:	Zuständige/r Pathologe/in:
Institutseigene Histoprotokollnummer:	

Lokalisation:	☐ Ösophagus	☐ Colon	Dignität:
	☐ Magen	☐ Rektum	☐ gutartig
	☐ Duodenum	☐ Leber	☐ bösartig
	☐ Jejunum	☐ Pankreas	☐ unklar
	☐ Ileum	☐ Kopf ☐ Körper ☐ Schwanz	Differenzierung:
	☐ Appendix	☐ Meckelsches Divertikel	☐ hoch differenziert
	☐ Spitze ☐ Basis	☐ Gallenblase	☐ niedrig differenziert

Multiple Endokrine Neoplasie I (MEN I): ☐ ja ☐ nein

A.4. Metastasen

Nachgewiesen: ☐ ja ☐ nein (weiter bei A.6)	
Lokalisation:	Anzahl
1.	
2.	
3.	
4.	
5.	

A.5 Weitere Krebserkrankungen

Vorhanden ☐ ja ☐ nein (weiter bei A.7)	
Genaue Diagnose :	Zeitpunkt d. Auftretens
1.	☐ synchron ☐ metachron davor ☐ metachron danach
2.	☐ synchron ☐ metachron davor ☐ metachron danach
3.	☐ synchron ☐ metachron davor ☐ metachron danach

A.6 Kommentar

Studienkennzahl:	Erfassungsdatum:

B Anamnese und Diagnostik

B.1 Klinische Untersuchung

Untersuchungsdatum:	
Größe:	Gewicht:
Symptome:	
☐ Muskelkrämpfe	☐ Flush
☐ Nachtschweiß	☐ Teleangieektasien
☐ Gewichtsverlust (kg in Wochen)	☐ Rechtsherzinsuffizienz
☐ Gewichtszunahme (kg in Wochen)	☐ Bronchospasmus
☐ Fieber	
☐ abdominelle Schmerzen	☐ Schwindel
☐ Diarrhö	☐ Bewusstlosigkeit
☐ Erbrechen	☐ neurologische Symptome
☐ Verstopfung	☐ Psychiatrische Auffälligkeit
☐ Hunger	☐ Krämpfe (epileptiform)
☐ Appetitverlust	☐ Schwitzen
☐ Diabetes mellitus	☐ Tremor
☐ Schwitzen	
☐ Aszites	☐ Magen-/Duodenalulcera
☐ Ikterus	(rezidivierend: ☐ ja ☐ nein)
☐ Ileus	☐ Gastroösophagealer Reflux
☐ Blut im Stuhl	
☐ Meläna	☐ Nekrotisierendes Erythema migrans
☐ Palpabler Tumor	
☐ Tiefe Venenthrombose	

B.2 Tumordiagnostik - Bildgebung

Technik	Durchgeführt	Datum	Nachweis:
MRT	☐ ja ☐ nein		☐ positiv ☐ negativ
CT	☐ ja ☐ nein		☐ positiv ☐ negativ
Ultraschall	☐ ja ☐ nein		☐ positiv ☐ negativ
Thorax-Röntgen	☐ ja ☐ nein		☐ positiv ☐ negativ
Endoskopischer Ultraschall	☐ ja ☐ nein		☐ positiv ☐ negativ
Somatostatin-Scan	☐ ja ☐ nein		☐ positiv ☐ negativ
PET-Scan Technik (Tracer):	☐ ja ☐ nein		☐ positiv ☐ negativ
Szintigraphie	☐ ja ☐ nein		☐ positiv ☐ negativ
Maximaler Durchmesser:			

B.3 Metastasendiagnostik - Bildgebung

Metastasen nachgewiesen: ☐ ja ☐ nein (weiter bei B.4)

Technik	Nachweis	Lokalisation	Anzahl	Max. Ø
MRT	☐ positiv ☐ negativ	1. 2. 3. 4.		
CT	☐ positiv ☐ negativ	1. 2. 3. 4.		
Ultraschall	☐ positiv ☐ negativ	1. 2. 3. 4.		

Studienkennzahl:	Erfassungsdatum:

Endoskopischer Ultraschall	☐ positiv ☐ negativ	1. 2. 3. 4.		
Nuklearmedizinische Diagnositk Typ:	☐ positiv ☐ negativ	1. 2. 3. 4.		

B.4 Labor

Spezielle Laboruntersuchungen für Neuroendokrine Tumore durchgeführt
☐ ja ☐ nein (weiter bei B.5)

Basalwerte		Sekretintest		Fastentest (Werte bei Beendigung)	
Chromogranin	µg/l	Gastrin (pg/ml)		Dauer in h:	
5-HIAA (Urin)	µmol/d	0 Min	pg/ml	Glukose:	mg/dl
Serotonin	ng/ml	2 Min	pg/ml	Insulin:	mE/l
Insulin	pmol/ml	5 Min	pg/ml	C-peptide	ng/ml
Glukagon	pg/ml	10 Min	pg/ml	Ausschluss von Sulfonylharnstoffen	☐ Ja ☐ Nein
Gastrin	pg/ml	15 Min	pg/ml		
VIP	pg/ml	30 Min	pg/ml		
NSE	µg/l				
Andere (Histamin, Somatostatin)					

B.5 Kommentar

Studienkennzahl:	Erfassungsdatum:

C Therapie

C.1 Endoskopische/Interventionelle Therapie (Polypabtragung, Stent etc.)

Durchgeführt ☐ ja ☐ nein (weiter bei C.2)
Abteilung:
Datum:
Operationstyp: ☐ kurativ ☐ palliativ ☐ Notfall ☐ andere:
OP-Technik:
Tumorgröße(n):
Durch Therapie geänderte histologische Diagnose: ☐ ja ☐ nein
Wenn ja: Neue Diagnose:

Dignität:	Differenzierung:
☐ gutartig	☐ hoch differenziert
☐ bösartig	☐ niedrig differenziert
☐ unklar	

C.2 Operative Therapie

Durchgeführt ☐ ja ☐ nein (weiter bei C.3)
Abteilung:
OP-Datum:
Operationstyp: ☐ kurativ ☐ palliativ ☐ Notfall ☐ andere:
OP-Technik:
Resektion Primum: ☐ R0 ☐ R1 ☐ R2 ☐ Rx
Tumorgröße(n):
Lebermetastasen: ☐ ja ☐ nein
Weitere Metastasen: ☐ ja ☐ nein
Resektion Metastasen: ☐ R0 ☐ R1 ☐ R2 ☐ Rx
Durch Therapie geänderte histologische Diagnose: ☐ ja ☐ nein
Wenn ja: Neue Diagnose:

Dignität:	Differenzierung:
☐ gutartig	☐ hoch differenziert
☐ bösartig	☐ niedrig differenziert
☐ unklar	

C.3 Ablations-Therapie

Durchgeführt ☐ ja ☐ nein (weiter bei C.4)
Abteilung:
Datum:
Technik: ☐ RFA (Radio-Frequenz Ablation)   ☐ Embolisation. Methodik (Chemo, Lipiodol, SIRT, etc.)   ☐ Kryotherapie   ☐ LITT (Laser-induced thermo therapy)   ☐ RRPT (Radio receptor peptid therapy).   Methodik (z.B. Y-DOTATOC, Lu-DOTATATE, etc.):

Studienkennzahl:	Erfassungsdatum:

C.4 Konservative Therapie
Durchgeführt ☐ ja ☐ nein (weiter bei D)

C.4.1 Somatostatin-Analoga-Therapie
Durchgeführt ☐ ja ☐ nein

Datum:	Medikament (Lanreotide, Octreotide etc.)	Applikation (s.c., i.a, Depot etc.)	Dosis + Anwendungsdauer	Abbruch wegen

C.4.2 Interferon
Durchgeführt ☐ ja ☐ nein

Datum:	Medikament (IF alfa-2b, Intron A, pegyliertes Interferon)	Applikation (s.c., i.a, Depot etc.)	Dosis + Anwendungsdauer	Abbruch wegen

C.4.3 Chemotherapie
Durchgeführt ☐ ja ☐ nein

Datum:	Medikament (Streptozocin, 5-FU etc.)	Dosis + Anzahl d. Zyklen	Abbruch wegen

C.5 Kommentar

Studienkennzahl:	Erfassungsdatum:

D Follow up
Patient steht/stand unter weiterer Kontrolle bzw. Behandlung ☐ ja   ☐ nein (Fragebogen beendet)

D.1 Klinik

Persistenz d. klinischen Symptome ☐ ja ☐ nein (weiter bei D.2)	
☐ Muskelkrämpfe	☐ Flush
☐ Nachtschweiß	☐ Teleangieektasien
☐ Gewichtsverlust (kg in Wochen)	☐ Rechtsherzinsuffizienz
☐ Gewichtszunahme (kg in Wochen)	☐ Bronchospasmus
☐ Fieber	
☐ abdominelle Schmerzen	☐ Schwindel
☐ Diarrhö	☐ Bewusstlosigkeit
☐ Erbrechen	☐ neurologische Symptome
☐ Verstopfung	☐ Psychiatrische Auffälligkeit
☐ Hunger	☐ Krämpfe (epileptiform)
☐ Appetitverlust	☐ Schwitzen
☐ Diabetes mellitus	☐ Tremor
☐ Schwitzen	
☐ Aszites	☐ Magen-/Duodenalulcera
☐ Ikterus	(rezidivierend: ☐ ja ☐ nein)
☐ Ileus	☐ Gastroösophagealer Reflux
☐ Blut im Stuhl	
☐ Meläna	☐ Nekrotisierendes Erythema migrans
☐ Palpabler Tumor	
☐ Tiefe Venenthrombose	

D.2 Verhalten des Primärtumors
D.2.1 Tumor Verhalten (gemäß RECIST-Kriterien)

☐ Stable disease   ☐ partial response   ☐ complete response   ☐ progressive diesease

D.2.2 Kontrolluntersuchungen

Technik	Durchgeführt	Datum
MRT	☐ ja ☐ nein	
CT	☐ ja ☐ nein	
Ultraschall	☐ ja ☐ nein	
Thorax-Röntgen	☐ ja ☐ nein	
Endoskopischer Ultraschall	☐ ja ☐ nein	
Somatostatin-Scan	☐ ja ☐ nein	
PET-Scan	☐ ja ☐ nein	
Technik (Tracer):		
Szintigraphie	☐ ja ☐ nein	
Maximaler Durchmesser:		

D.2.3 Weitere Metastasierung

Nachgewiesen: ☐ ja ☐ nein (weiter bei D.3)		
Lokalisation	Anzahl	Max. Durchmesser
1.		
2.		
3.		

Studienkennzahl:	Erfassungsdatum:

D.3 Verlauf der Laborparameter

Spezielle Laborverlaufskontrolle durchgeführt: ☐ ja ☐ nein		
	Datum	Wert
Chromogranin A:		
Hormon:		

D.4 Kommentar

8.5 Appendix E: Approval

Approval of the ethics committee of the Medical University of Vienna (Resolution number 157/2005).

**ETHIK-KOMMISSION
DER MEDIZINISCHEN UNIVERSITÄT WIEN
UND DES
ALLGEMEINEN KRANKENHAUSES DER STADT WIEN AKH**
Borschkegasse 8b/6 - A-1090 Wien, Austria
☎ 0043 1 404 00 – 2147 & 📠 0043 1 404 00 – 1690
E-Mail: ethik-kom@meduniwien.ac.at
www.univie.ac.at/ethik-kom

Sitzung der Ethikkommission am 9. Mai 2005, TOP 41 :

EK Nr: 157/2005
Antragsteller: Univ.Prof.Dr. Bruno Niederle
Einreichende Institution: Univ.Klin.f. Chirurgie
Projekttitel: Gastroenteropankreatische Neuroendokrine Tumore (GEP-NET)

Die Stellungnahme der Ethik-Kommission erfolgt aufgrund folgender eingereichter Unterlagen:

Dokument	Version/Nr	Datiert
Originalprotokoll: GEP-NET		undatiert
Kurzfassung:		undatiert
Patienteninfo./Einverständniserklrg.:		undatiert

Die Kommission faßt folgenden Beschluß (mit X markiert):

☒ Es besteht kein Einwand gegen die Durchführung der Studie.

☐ Die unten bezeichneten Punkte des Antrages sind entweder noch unerledigt bzw sollten von den Antragstellern geändert/ nachgereicht werden. Nach entsprechender Vorlage/Erledigung kann auch vor der nächsten Ethik-Kommissions Sitzung ein endgültig positiver Beschluß ausgefertigt werden. Der Antrag wird in der nächsten Sitzung der Kommission nicht mehr behandelt.
Achtung: Werden die geforderten Unterlagen von den Antragstellern nicht innerhalb von 3 Sitzungsperioden (ab Datum dieser Sitzung) nachgereicht, gilt der Antrag ohne weitere Benachrichtigung als zurückgezogen und muß gegebenenfalls als Neuantrag eingereicht werden.

☐ Es bestehen Einwände gegen die Durchführung der Studie in der eingereichten Form. Die unten angeführten Punkte sollten von den Antragstellern entsprechend geändert und der Kommission neu vorgelegt werden. Der Antrag wird in der nächsten Sitzung der Kommission nochmals behandelt.
Achtung: Werden die geforderten Unterlagen von den Antragstellern nicht innerhalb von 3 Sitzungsperioden (ab Datum dieser Sitzung) nachgereicht, gilt der Antrag ohne weitere Benachrichtigung als zurückgezogen und muß gegebenenfalls als Neuantrag eingereicht werden.

☐ Der Antrag wird von der Ethik-Kommission abgelehnt.

☐ Der TOP wird bis zur nächsten Sitzung vertagt (Begründung siehe unten)

Kommentare:

Zum Prüfplan :

Zur Patienteninformation :

Zur Versicherungsbestätigung : **nicht erforderlich**

Andere :

Die Ethik-Kommission geht - rechtlich unverbindlich – davon aus, daß es sich um keine klinische Prüfung gemäß AMG/MPG handelt.

Mitgliederliste der Ethik-Kommission (aktueller Stand am Sitzungstag) beiliegend. Mitglieder der Ethik-Kommission, die für diesen Tagesordnungspunkt als befangen anzusehen waren und daher laut Geschäftsordnung an der Entscheidungsfindung/Abstimmung nicht teilgenommen haben: **Dr. Michael Gnant**

Univ.Prof.Dr. Ernst Singer
Vorsitzender der Kommission

ACHTUNG: Unter Berücksichtigung der „ICH-Guideline for Good Clinical Practice" gilt dieser Beschluß **ein Jahr ab Datum der Ausstellung.** Gegebenenfalls hat der Antragsteller eine Verlängerung der Gültigkeit mittels Formular für „Meldungen" rechtzeitig vorzulegen.

9. Lists

9.1 List of abbreviations

^{111}In	111 - Indium
^{177}Lu	177 - Lutetium
5-FU	5-Fluoruracil
5HT	5-Hydroxytryptamine
^{90}Y	90 - Yttrium
ACTH	Adrenocorticotropic hormone
AD	Anno domini
AJCC	American Joint Cancer Committee
APUD	Amine precursor uptake and decarboxylation
ATP	Adenosintriphosphat
BC	Before christ
bHLH	Basic helix loop helix
Ca	Calcium
CAG	Chronic atrophic gastritis
CALC	Calcitonin-gene-related peptide
cAMP	Cyclic adenosinmonophosphate
CCK	Cholecystokinin
CgA	Chromogranin A
CGH	Comparative genomic hybridization
CK	Cytokeratin
CNS	Central nervous system
cox	Cytochrom c oxidase deficiency
CRGP	Calcitonin-gene-related peptide
CT	Computed tomography
DNA	Desoxyribonucleic acid
DCC	Deleted in Colorectal Cancer (gene)
DOTA	1,4,7,10-tetraazacyclododecane-1,4,7,10-tetraacetic acid
DOTA-TATE	DOTA Octreotate
DTPA	Diethylene triamine pentaacetic acid
DTPA-OC	DTPA - Octreotide
EC	Enterochromaffin cell
ecl	Enterochromaffin-like cell
EGF	Endothelic growth factor
ENETS	European neuroendocrine tumours society
ENS	Enteric nervous system
EUS	Endoscopical ultrasound
FGF	Fibroblastic growth factor
G6PD	Glucose-6-phosphate dehydrogenase
GABA	Gamma amino butyric acid
GEP	Gastro-entero pancreatic
GHRH	Growth hormone releasing hormone
GHS-R	Growth hormone secretagogue receptor
Gi	G inhibiting
GIP	Gastric inhibitory polypeptide or Glucose dependent insulinotropic polypeptide
GLP	Glucagon like protein

GRP	Gastrin releasing peptide
hes	Hairy and enhancer of split
HIF	Hypoxia-inducible factor
hox	Homebox
HPF	High power field
IFN	Interferon
IGF	Insulin-like growth factor
IGFBP3	Insulin-like-growth-factor-binding-protein 3
IQR	Interquartile range
ki-67	Kiel-67
K-Ras	V-Ki-ras2 = Kirsten rat sarcoma viral oncogene homo
LAR	Long-acting repeatable
LDCV	Large dense core vesicles
LOH	Loss of heterozygosity
MANEC	Mixed adenoneuroendocrine carcinoma
MAO	Monoamine-oxidase
MEN	Multiple endocrine neoplasia
MIB-1	Monoclonal antibody-1
MMC	Migrating motor complex
MRI	Magnetic Resonance Imaging
MRT	Magnetic resonance tomography
N-CAM	Neural cell adhesion molecules
NCI	National Cancer institute
NE	Neuroendocrine
NET	Neuroendocrine tumour
NF-1	Neurofibromatosis type 1
ngn	Neurogenin
NO	Nitric oxide
NOS	Not otherwise specified
NPY	Neuropetide Y
NSE	Neuron specific enolase
NSF	N-ethylmaleimide-sensitive factor
p53	Protein 53
PACAP	Pituitary adenylat cyclase activating peptide
pax	Paired box
PC	Proprotein convertase
pdx1	Pyridoxal
PET	Positron emission tomography
PET-CT	Positron emission tomography computed tomography
PGP 9.5	Protein gene product 9.5
PHI	Peptide histamine isoleucin
PHM	Peptide histidine methionine
PHM	Peptide histidine methionine
PNETS	Pancreatic neuroendocrine tumours
PP	Pancreatic polypetide
PRRT	Peptide-receptor-radio-therapy
PTEN	Phosphatase and tensin homolog
pTNM	Postoperative TNM
PYY	Peptide YY
RER	Rough endoplasmatic reticulum

RNA	Ribonucleic acid
SEER	Surveillance, Epidemiology and End result
SLMV	Synaptic-like microvesicles
SNARE	Soluble NSF-associated attachment receptor
SS	Somatostatin
SSA	Somatostatin analogue
SSTR	Somatostatin receptro
SSV	Small synaptic vesicles
SV	Synaptic vesicle protein
Syn	Synaptophysin
TACE	Trans-catheter arterial chemoembolisation
TAE	Trans-catheter arterial embolisation
TGF	Transforming growth factor
Tis	Tumour in situ
TLL	Tumour-like lesions
TNCS	Third National Cancer Survey
TNM	Tumour/Noduli/Metastases
TRH	Thyrotropin-releasing hormone
UICC	Union Internationale Contre le Cancer
USA	United States of America
VHL	Von-Hippel-Lindau
VIP	Vasoactive intestinal peptide
VMAT	Vesicular monoamine transporter
VPAC	Vasoactive intestinal peptide/pituitary adenylate cyclase-activating polypeptide type
WHO	World health organisation
WWII	World War 2
ZES	Zollinger Ellison syndrome

9.2 List of tables

Table 1 - GI neuroendocrine cell types, their localisations and main products (after [33, 34]) 30

Table 2 - Classification of neuroendocrine tumors of the gastroenteropancreatic system (GEP-NET); adapted after [62] 48

Table 3 - Criteria for assessing the prognosis of neuroendocrine tumours of the intestine [62, 63] 49

Table 4 - Criteria for assessing the prognosis of neuroendocrine tumours of the pancreas [62, 63] 49

Table 5 - Comparison of the WHO 2000 and the WHO 2010 classification of neuroendocrine neoplasms of the digestive system (after [69]) 50

Table 6 - Proposal for a grading system for neuroendocrine tumours [70, 71] 51

Table 7 - Overview about the classification of neuroendocrine tumours of the stomach; taken from [62] 55

Table 8 - Proposal for a pTNM classification for neuroendocrine tumours of the stomach; taken from [70, 72] 56

Table 9 - Proposal for disease staging for neuroendocrine tumours of the stomach; taken from [77] 57

Table 10 - Overview about the classification of neuroendocrine tumours of the duodenum and upper jejunum; taken from [62] 59

Table 11 - Proposal for a pTNM classification for neuroendocrine tumours of the duodenum/ampulla/jejunum and ileum; adapted from [70, 72] 60

Table 12 - Proposal for disease staging for neuroendocrine tumours of the duodenum/ampulla/jejunum and ileum; adapted from [77] 61

Table 13 - Overview about the classification of neuroendocrine tumours of the pancreas; taken from [62] 66

Table 14 - Proposal for a pTNM classification for neuroendocrine tumours of the pancreas; taken from [71, 72] 67

Table 15 - Proposal for disease staging by ENETS for neuroendocrine tumours of the pancreas; taken from [77] 67

Table 16 – Proposal for disease staging by AJCC/UICC for neuroendocrine tumours of the pancreas; taken from [72] 68

Table 17 - Overview of the classification of neuroendocrine tumours of the ileum, cecum, colon and rectum; taken from [62] 70

Table 18 - Proposal for a pTNM classification for neuroendocrine tumours of the duodenum/ampulla/jejunum and ileum; adapted from [71, 72] 71

Table 19 - Proposal for disease staging for neuroendocrine tumours of the duodenum/ampulla/jejunum and ileum; adapted from [77] 72

Table 20 - Overview of the classification of neuroendocrine tumours of the appendix; taken from [62] 74

Table 21 - Proposal for a pTNM classification for neuroendocrine tumours of the appendix; taken from [71, 72] 75

Table 22 - Proposal for disease staging by ENETS of neuroendocrine tumours of the appendix; taken from [77] 76

Table 23 – Proposal for disease staging by AJCC/UICC of neuroendocrine tumours of the appendix, taken from [72] 76

Table 24 - Proposal for a pTNM classification of neuroendocrine tumours of the colon and rectum; taken from [71, 72] 78

Table 25 - Proposal for disease staging of neuroendocrine tumours of the colon and rectum; taken from [77] 79

Table 26 - Age-adjusted incidence rates* n/100000/year for the white US-population for the years 1950-69[97] 91

Table 27 – Age adjusted incidence rates* n/100000/year for the white US-population for the years 1992-1999 92

Table 28 – Age-adjusted* incidence rates n/100000/year for the Swedish population for the years 1983-1998. * No information about which standard population was used 93

Table 29 – Age-adjusted standardised incidence rates* n/100000/year for Canton Vaud, Switzerland for the years 1974-1997 94

Table 30 - Site and incidence of malignant neuroendocrine tumours and other malignancies of the digestive tract 115

Table 31 - ENETS staging based on details of 181 of 277 (65.3%) patients 116

Table 32 - Comparison of WHO 2000 [63] and WHO 2010 [69] using the example of 77 (27.8%) of 277 NETs documented within this clinical investigation 135

Table 33 - Diagnosing department, diagnostic procedures, and incidental diagnosis of neuroendocrine tumors 136

Table 34 - Treatment modalities in patients with neuroendocrine tumors: surgery, endoscopy, no intervention 137

Table 35 - Endoscopic and surgical interventions in 188 patients in relation to WHO 2000 classification and NET location 138

Table 36 - Location of metastasis: 104/277 (37.5%) tumors classified as malignant (WHO 2 and 3) using the WHO criteria 139

Table 37 - Additional malignancy: clinical data available in 176/277 (61.7%) patients with neuroendocrine tumors 140

Table 38 - Medical treatment of patients with neuroendocrine tumors 141

9.3 List of figures

Figure 1 - Schematic and simplified phylogenetic tree adapted from S. Leach [29] 21

Figure 2 – Study algorithm 96

Figure 3 - Number (%), location and biological behaviour of neuroendocrine tumours in each site 117

Figure 4 - Malignant neuroendocrine tumours of the digestive tract – well-differentiated and poorly-differentiated neuroendocrine carcinoma 118

Figure 5 - Incidence rates of GEP neuroendocrine tumours (n/100,000/year); age-adjusted using the US 2000 standard population comparing the recent data with Norway and the USA [107] 119

Figure 6 - Incidence rates of GEP neuroendocrine tumours (n/100,000/year); age-adjusted using the world standard population comparing the recent data with Sweden [99] and Switzerland [100] 120

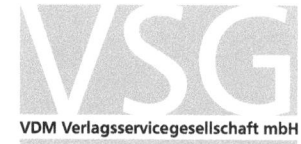

VDM Verlagsservicegesellschaft mbH

Die VDM Verlagsservicegesellschaft sucht für wissenschaftliche Verlage abgeschlossene und herausragende

Dissertationen, Habilitationen, Diplomarbeiten, Master Theses, Magisterarbeiten usw.

für die kostenlose Publikation als Fachbuch.

Sie verfügen über eine Arbeit, die hohen inhaltlichen und formalen Ansprüchen genügt, und haben Interesse an einer honorarvergüteten Publikation?

Dann senden Sie bitte erste Informationen über sich und Ihre Arbeit per Email an *info@vdm-vsg.de*.

Sie erhalten kurzfristig unser Feedback!

VDM Verlagsservicegesellschaft mbH
Dudweiler Landstr. 99   Telefon +49 681 3720 174
D - 66123 Saarbrücken   Fax   +49 681 3720 1749
www.vdm-vsg.de

Die VDM Verlagsservicegesellschaft mbH vertritt

 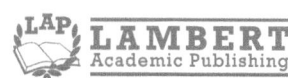 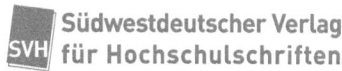

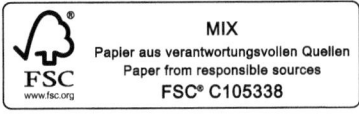

Printed by Books on Demand GmbH, Norderstedt / Germany